In the Kingdom of the Sick

Life Disrupted: Getting Real About Chronic Illness in Your Twenties and Thirties

IN THE KINGDOM OF THE SICK

A SOCIAL HISTORY OF CHRONIC
ILLNESS IN AMERICA

Laurie Edwards

Walker & Company
New York

Published by Walker Publishing Company, Inc., New York
A Division of Bloomsbury Publishing

All papers used by Walker & Company are natural, recyclable products made
from wood grown in well-managed forests. The manufacturing processes
conform to the environmental regulations of the country of origin.

LIBRARY OF CONGRESS CATALOGING-IN-PUBLICATION DATA HAS BEEN APPLIED FOR.

ISBN: 978-0-8027-1801-3

Visit Walker & Company's website at www.walkerbooks.com

First U.S. edition 2013

1   3   5   7   9   10   8   6   4   2

Typeset by Westchester Book Group
Printed in the United States by Thomson-Shore, Inc., Dexter, Michigan

For Victoria,
my joy

Contents

Introduction

WHEN I was growing up in the 1980s and '90s, Boston's famed Longwood Medical Area was as much my place of education as the small parochial grammar school I attended. Some of my most vivid memories were of my mother driving me down Route 9 to my doctor appointments, past the strip malls and chain restaurants of the western suburbs, past the reservoir in Brookline, where the crimson autumn leaves formed a circle around the gray expanse of water. These morning drives are almost always sunny and autumnal in my memory; we would squint up as we were stopped at traffic lights, always worried about being a little late, always underestimating the drive or underestimating our likelihood of getting every red light through three or four towns.

If it was a good appointment, I'd leave with an antibiotic script for my ever-present ear and sinus infections, a follow-up appointment, or a referral for yet another specialist for my wheezy lungs. If it was a bad appointment, it would usually involve a CT scan, a blood test, or the scheduling of another surgery. Either way, we'd get in the car and head back down Route 9, usually too late for me to make it back to school—I knew this would happen but wore my uniform anyway—but just early enough to beat rush-hour traffic. We would talk about my upcoming surgery, or about the books I would get as presents for my recovery, or the classes I'd missed and the sleepover I hoped I'd make it to on the weekend.

But chronic illness? I don't remember hearing that term, and I certainly don't remember using it in reference to my own patient experiences. I lived in reaction to each illness event, never quite acknowledging the larger pattern.

It wasn't just another infection, another setback, another disruption. *It wasn't going to go away.*

Certainly, I don't blame the grade school version of myself for overlooking this distinction, or the high school and college version, either. Even if I knew it intellectually by then, emotionally it was another adjustment altogether. And I know I wasn't alone. In fact, I think this is the most daunting aspect of any chronic illness, whether you are the patient grappling with a diagnosis or a healthy person who hopes it never happens to you: It isn't going to go away.

Back then, I was a kid who was sick, who divided her time between school, friends and family, and doctors and hospitals. Now, I am an adult patient with lung and autoimmune diseases: primary ciliary dyskinesia (PCD), bronchiectasis, and celiac disease, among other conditions. I cough and wheeze a lot, and since I don't have the working cilia to flush out mucus and debris from my lungs and respiratory tract, I get a lot of infections that compromise my airways and my oxygenation. I have daily chest physical therapy, in which my lung lobes are "clapped" in several different positions. I take pills for a sluggish thyroid and use inhalers and nebulizers to help keep my airways open, and long-term antibiotics are a necessary evil in my world. I've spent far too many weeks of my life in the hospital, including the trauma unit and the ICU, but I've also done so much of what healthy people do: graduated high school and college; studied abroad for a year; pursued a graduate degree; and got married. I spent four long years trying to have a child and made it through a medically intensive, complicated pregnancy to deliver a healthy little girl. I work full time and have freelance work. These are the extremes that characterize life with chronic illness, and almost 130 million Americans contend with them to some degree.[1]

Much about chronic illness has changed since I was a child. People with cystic fibrosis, a disease similar to my own lung disease, have seen their life expectancy reach almost forty, and people with type 1 diabetes can use insulin pumps and continuous glucose monitors to control their blood sugar instead of relying on shots. It is now a mandate that clinical research trials include women and minorities, and the thorny relationship between pain and gender is discussed more widely.[2] Children now spend more time watching television or using computers than playing outside, and First Lady Michelle Obama launched a campaign to fight against childhood obesity. Patients can e-mail their doctors and get text messages from their pharmacies, and social media platforms are now places where patients connect and advocate.

It is a whole different world, indeed. Cultural, scientific, political, and economic influences have changed how we classify and respond to the patient with chronic illness. Centuries ago, disease was thought to stem from an imbalance of bodily humors and fluids; infectious plagues were blamed on divine retribution; people with tuberculosis were shipped off to sanatoriums; and diseases like multiple sclerosis were considered nervous or hysterical disorders. In more recent decades past, chronic illness conjured images of arthritic elderly patients, and cancer was still spoken of in metaphors and hushed tones, which Susan Sontag assailed in her polemic *Illness as Metaphor.*

When the idea for this book first took root several years ago, I was a young college English instructor teaching a debut course called "Constructions of Health in Contemporary Literature" to a group of college freshman interested in the health sciences. As we tackled such heavyweights as David B. Morris and Sontag, I worried about relevancy. Would my students see the connections between illness and culture, between the words we use to describe and assimilate illness and the actual patient experience? They might not have been as intrigued or riled up by the use of metaphorical language as I was, but relevancy was not something I needed to worry about, after all. They spoke of loved ones with cancer, and of depression and addiction. They were riveted by *Frontline's Age of AIDS* documentary, and wondered how proceeds from the red Razr phones they saw advertised would really play into AIDS research, as the holiday commercials they watched touted. They saw the blurring of consumption, culture, and sickness, and they realized that the science they learned in other classes did not exist in the vacuum of the classroom or the laboratory.

In 1999 the scholar and medical historian Roy Porter asserted, "Disease is a social development no less than the medicine that combats it."[3] Porter's claim is equally germane today, even though, as my students and I discovered, the stakes have changed. Now, for as much knowledge as we have about the biological origins of many genetic, autoimmune, and viral disorders, still millions live with illnesses that aren't merely "invisible" to others but are not easily identified in laboratories or imaging centers, either. For as many technological and lifestyle resources as we have at our disposal, for as "good" as our health is compared to centuries past, larger numbers of us are sick.

"The medical arena is just a microcosm of society in general," says Dr. Sarah Whitman, a psychiatrist specializing in the treatment of chronic pain, one of the most common and debilitating manifestations of chronic illness. The tensions surrounding sex, gender, socioeconomic status, and power that dominate our cultural consciousness are the same ones so instrumental to the emergence of chronic illness as social phenomenon. While female patients with CFIDS (chronic fatigue and immune dysfunction syndrome) are told their symptoms are the somatic manifestations of upper-middle-class social anxiety, patients with diseases as varied as HIV or type 2 diabetes labor under their own stigmas: that they are responsible for their preventable illnesses and that their lifestyle choices are subject to judgment by others. And of course, the rampant health disparities between rich and poor are drawn out in spectacularly dramatic fashion when it comes to chronic disease: fewer resources and less access to care equals less prevention, more disease progression, and a whole host of confluent problems. On the Internet and on television and radio programs, political debates about health care reform continue to rage on.

So how do we begin to unravel all of this?

Thirty years ago Susan Sontag famously wrote, "Illness is the night-side of life, a more onerous citizenship. Everyone who is born holds dual citizenship, in the kingdom of the well and the kingdom of the sick . . . sooner or later each of us is obliged, at least for a spell, to identify ourselves as citizens of that other place."[4] As the scope of chronic conditions continues to widen, Sontag's distinction is even more poignant. The statisticians and experts tell us that more and more of us do—or will—belong to that "other place." For one, we live longer and have more interventional therapies available so we accumulate inevitable ailments of aging. For another, those with serious diseases have better diagnostics and treatments, meaning they too are living longer into adulthood with serious illness. On the whole, our lifestyle shifts also play a role in the irritatingly named "diseases of affluence." Western society not only cultivates but exports cancer, obesity, coronary heart disease, hypertension, type 2 diabetes, and other chronic conditions to developing nations.[5]

As it did with the infectious and communicable diseases of the past, science is responsible for un-shrouding the mysteries of chronic illness. In some cases, it has; but in many others, the competing forces of fear, guilt, and shame blur the clarifications science supposedly offers us. A gap still exists between the potential of science and technology to answer questions about disease and the social constructs we erect around notions of what it means to be ill.

From online forums and patient blogs to social media, direct-to-consumer marketing of pharmaceuticals, and consumer health privacy concerns, technology asserts itself into the patient experience in numerous ways. For example, we can trade stories and swap advice; we can push for research or work to increase awareness of little-known disorders. Vaccinations against communicable diseases represent some of modern medicine's greatest triumphs, yet perhaps nowhere has the sharing of anecdotal patient stories had more impact than in the controversy over childhood vaccinations. Here, the power of the patient activist and new media is pitted against the established institutional authority of medicine, and just how this battle plays out will have profound consequences for us all.

As a health and science writer, I see trends like individual responsibility for behavior versus random chance or genetic mutations, consumption versus philanthropy, and the basic working definitions of what is "healthy" versus what is "sick" through the prism of journal articles and analysis. As a lifelong patient with multiple chronic illnesses, I see the physical realities of chronic illness as well as their emotional implications. Every day, I wake up, feed my child, take my medications, and put on the trappings of the well. I am her mother, first and foremost, and that does not change depending on my symptoms.

In front of a classroom of students or on the phone with a freelance client, I might be many things, but I am not sick. Even if they hear my hacking cough or notice the dark circles under my eyes, they do not know the reality of what goes on behind my front door, or in my doctor's office or a hospital room. I am used to such deceiving appearances, and I depend on technology to keep up the façade when I need it.

On days when I feel worse, it is an active, deliberate choice to enter Sontag's kingdom of the well, just as it is sometimes a conscious act to breathe, to focus on the rhythms of *inhale* and *exhale* and not the chortling wheezes and sticky congestion that make those motions so challenging. I am not alone in this daily negotiation, and beyond the numbers are the compromises and compensations made by all people living with some form of chronic condition.

In the Kingdom of the Sick is a combination of research, literature, and stories from patients across the chronic disease spectrum. Literary inspiration comes from many sources, from Katherine Anne Porter's tale of the post–World War One influenza pandemic, "Pale Horse, Pale Rider"— which I first read in high school—to *A Life in Medicine*, a compilation edited by Dr. Robert Coles and others that includes fiction and nonfiction tales of treating patients, of living with illness, of fear, beauty, and mortality. The rich contents of *A Life in Medicine* piqued my interest while I was a graduate student and fledgling instructor. Books by Andrew Solomon, Paula Kamen, Roy Porter, David Rothman, and many, many others made me start asking questions.

- What does it mean for patients that the definition of chronic illness is fairly static but its scope has changed so much?
- How will long-standing gender biases in the treatment and diagnosis of pain shift if we find more evidence to support biological differences between how women and men experience pain?
- How will technology change the doctor-patient relationship, and how will technology empower patients?

- Will patients with chronic illness ever see the type of focused mobilization that made the disability and HIV/AIDS movements a success?
- And, as Roy Porter queried, if disease is a social development as much as its treatments are, what will the experience of living with chronic illness be like as we move forward?

In a way, I see these writers as specialists, people who have focused on one topic (pain, disability, gender, cancer, autoimmune disease, etc.) masterfully. In writing about chronic illness, I am an inevitable generalist, someone who is pulling ideas together and looking at larger patterns among them in a different way. As such, *In the Kingdom of the Sick* is a big-picture book, focusing less on disease-specific symptoms and more on the universal aspects of the circumstances in which illness unfolds.

Though it is not a uniform linear history of disease, *In the Kingdom of the Sick* does focus primarily on the decades following World War Two, decades in which science, politics, and social justice all converged in such a way as to leave a lasting, transformative impression on the illness experience. I am not a sociologist, a historian, a physician, or a legal scholar. I am a lifelong patient with chronic illness who has always had health insurance, who has had access to some of the best hospitals in the world, and who nonetheless spent much of her life as a medical mystery within those hallowed institutions. Like it or not, I will take medication and have chest physical therapy for the rest of my life. I will never know what it is to be "healthy," but I have learned that it is not worth the time and energy to lament or miss something you never had. I blog about chronic illness, I e-mail my doctors and log medical data on my iPhone, and it is only through technology that I have spoken to or met anyone else with my rare disease, PCD.

As one of my interviewees, e-Patient Dave deBronkart, described it, today's health care system is like a mobile with billions of pieces spinning around. Pulling at a thread will shift the other pieces around in a way that is complex and hard to predict. That analogy is at play in the chronic illness experience. Health care reform, direct-to-consumer pharmaceutical advertising, the influence of the environment and chemical exposure, so-cioeconomics, gender, politics, etc.—are all threads from the mobile, and each is interconnected to other threads. Here is where I stop pulling, stand still, and reflect on the threads that resonate most with me as a writer and as a patient with chronic illness.

If, as David B. Morris says, illness tells us more about an era or an individual than health does, we now find ourselves at an intersection, lodged between the promise of science and technology and lingering assumptions about people who are forced to dwell in the kingdom of the sick. What will their future look like? To hazard a guess, we must probe where attitudes about chronic illness came from, and where they stand today.

CHAPTER 1

From Plato to Polio
Chronic Disease in Historical Context

THIRTY-YEAR-OLD Melissa McLaughlin remembers in painstaking detail when she first became sick. It was late October 1994, and the then high school sophomore's crammed schedule reflected an active, passionate teenager: Advanced Placement courses, dance classes and competitions, the dance classes she taught to younger students, babysitting her siblings, volunteering. As a competitive dancer, she depended on her body to keep up with her rigorous schedule, and it always had.

"Everything was normal," she says.

The weeks building up to the seismic shift that would turn the energetic teenager into a wheelchair-bound young woman living in constant pain were normal, if hectic. She threw a Halloween party for the dance students she taught, and sat for the PSATs. Her last "normal" day was spent with friends painting the walls of a homeless shelter. By the day's end, the whole group was sweaty, exhausted, and covered in paint.

"All of us were worn out, but I just never got better," McLaughlin says, describing how she went to sleep that night and woke up with a high fever and extreme fatigue and body aches. For the first few weeks, she slept twenty-two hours a day, and her doctors initially diagnosed her with mononucleosis. At this point, she, like her doctors and most people around her, figured with a few more weeks of rest, she would be fine. That was how an acute condition like mono worked: you got it, you lived through it for a few weeks, and then it went away. Case closed. For many people, this is the trajectory we associate with illness. We are familiar with both ends of the spectrum: the short, acute infections and injuries of everyday life and the terminal cases of cancer, heart disease, or stroke that have a finite end. Chronic illness is somewhere in the middle, confounding and unfamiliar.

Weeks and months went by, and McLaughlin's improvement was minimal at best. She still slept several hours each day, only dragging herself into class half-days and often fainting when she was there. She could barely walk but tried to attend dance class anyway, only to fall asleep on a pile of mats in the corner. Her blood tests came back abnormal but not definitive, and as the months went on a variety of diagnoses were handed to her: chronic mono, Epstein-Barr virus, chronic fatigue syndrome (CFS), chronic fatigue and immune dysfunction syndrome (CFIDS). For each she was told there were no treatments, and the approach was reactive, treating symptoms and not causes. If she caught an infection—which was a regular occurrence—she was given antibiotics. If she had severe migraines, physicians prescribed migraine medication. When her extreme fatigue become even more overwhelming, they told her to get more rest. No one could explain how to make her better, and, just as frustratingly, no one could explain to her what had made her sick in the first place.

While the details vary, her physical manifestations and diagnostic roadblocks could stand in for the experience of millions of Americans over the past few decades. The history of CFS/CFIDS and related "nebulous" conditions in this country is a controversial one; even now, consensus over its name is lacking, and although many advocates of the disease fight for education and awareness, detractors remain. In *Encounters with the Invisible*, CFS patient Dorothy Wall calls the condition "so blatantly unmedicalized, so subjective, another one of those so-called 'functional illnesses,' like irritable bowel syndrome, that have always plagued medical practitioners, presenting symptoms with no known cause."[1] From dissent over labels and diagnostic categories to research dollars and clinical trials, the combination of politics, science, and policy is a potent one.

In *All in My Head*, Paula Kamen focuses on the other phenomenon at play, one as relevant and entrenched in attitudes today as it was in centuries past: If you cannot cure the patient, then blaming the patient often follows suit. When we don't understand the source of the problem or how we can alleviate it, "the more psychological, spiritual, and moral meaning it takes on."[2] History reveals the foundation of this current pattern, as we will see, but when physicians adopt this mindset, it is particularly harmful. In comparing nineteenth-century tuberculosis and late-twentieth-century cancer, Susan Sontag wrote, "Any disease that is treated as a mystery and acutely enough feared will be felt to be morally, if not literally, contagious."[3]

This applies to chronic illness, too. We do not like being reminded that there are still limits to modern medicine, and that named conditions exist that might not kill us but will not go away. But if we add to this scenario those illnesses that we can't name or file under International Statistical Classification of Diseases and Related Health Problems (ICD-10) codes on medical billing forms, conditions we can't put under our high-powered microscopes or see on advanced imaging tests, then the fear—and, often, distaste—grows. Perhaps if the symptoms can be explained away by claiming the patient is just lazy, or is not making appropriate lifestyle changes, then blame can replace the other niggling emotion: *Maybe if it can happen to him or her, it could happen to me.*

And likely, it will happen to many people at some point in their life. Chronic illness affects nearly 50 percent of the population. By the year 2025, it is estimated that chronic illness will affect some 164 million Americans.[4] Some of the most common are heart disease, diabetes, cancer, and asthma, but that list is by no means exhaustive. Arthritis, lupus, multiple sclerosis, Crohn's disease, colitis, epilepsy, and thousands of other diseases cause ongoing symptoms and are treatable but not curable. Chronic illness is the leading cause of death and disability in this country, with seven out of every ten deaths attributed to chronic diseases. Eighty-one percent of hospital admissions are a result of chronic illness, as are 76 percent of all physician visits. These statistics come with a hefty price tag, too; 75 percent of a staggering $2 trillion in health care costs in 2005 came from chronic diseases.

As the years passed, there was no doubt that Melissa McLaughlin dwelled in the kingdom of the sick. Her conditions weren't going away, and they caused ongoing quality-of-life problems and disability. Gradually, some of her diagnoses got more specific: the combination of CFIDS and fibromyalgia explained the fatigue and the pain. Postural orthostatic tachycardia syndrome (POTS), a dysregulation of the autonomic nervous system that interferes with heart rate and other functions, explained the fainting and cardiac issues. Neurally mediated hypotension (NMH), an inability to regulate blood pressure often found in patients with CFIDS, and hypogammaglobulinemia, which increases the risk of infection, were also added to the list.

However, if she thought that since she now had many labels and acronyms attached to her symptoms the skepticism of others she encountered toward her pain or her treatment options would improve significantly, she was mistaken.

"I had a friend once who said that my illnesses were the hippest thing about me. I'm no trendsetter, but I had CFIDS before it was cool, according to him," she says, aware of the antipathy that still surrounds the diagnosis of CFIDS. "Some doctors still sniff at the CFIDS/FM diagnoses, call them trash-barrel diagnoses. I say, that's fine, but unless you know what it really is, then you're not really helping anything, are you?" she asks.

And therein lies one of the most compelling tensions history reveals: the quest to understand the nature of illness from a biological perspective versus the quest to understand illness from a personal perspective.

For Emerson Miller, a forty-eight-year-old who is HIV-positive, his experience of illness has been no less challenging than Melissa McLaughlin's. Where chronic pain conditions and autoimmune disorders often prove difficult to isolate, the test for HIV/AIDS is all too definitive. Fifteen years ago, after Miller had suffered from a flu-like illness that left him seriously ill, doctors tested him and found an incredibly high viral load. It was the mid-1990s, and doctors were flush with excitement over the newly approved triple drug cocktail used to treat HIV/AIDS, though no one knew the long-term effects of the drugs and back then, incorrect dosing was still a significant problem. At the time of his diagnosis, this barely registered.

"I was so ill that I didn't care, I didn't care if I had three weeks to live," he says. It was a very different dynamic than the immediate experience of those patients who may feel okay but choose to get tested because of known risk factors or disclosure of illness from present or past partners. Miller recognizes this distinction acutely; in his job as a patient coordinator and advocate at AIDS Action Committee of Massachusetts in Boston, he witnesses firsthand the process of diagnosis, acceptance, and ongoing treatment of this next generation of HIV patients. The population is far more diverse now than it was in the early days of the "gay plague"—IV drug users, young heterosexual patients, and an increasing number of African-American and Hispanic females are just some of the groups who join homosexuals as sub-populations with very different needs—but some things remain the same. Despite many permutations, the stigma associated with HIV/AIDS and more specifically with the means of transmission that has characterized the HIV/AIDS epidemic since its beginning is still a predominant theme in living with the disease. It isn't simply a matter of prevailing societal norms of the healthy versus the sick that many of us experience. Miller describes an intricate hierarchy of blame or perhaps judgment, too: gay people are better than drug users, while hemophiliacs and those whose illnesses can't be attributed to lifestyle are innocent.

I often see a related form of hierarchy when it comes to suffering: patients who are quick to claim that their pain and "battle scars" are worse than those of other patients are an unfortunate reality in waiting rooms, support groups, and Internet forums. Both scenarios create internal divisions that weaken one of the greatest assets patients have in a healthy world: the solidarity of the illness experience.

"There is still a lot of shame about homosexuality. Even at my age . . . there is still a lot of shame," Miller says. "In my opinion, everybody is still a patient."

The dismissal, skepticism, and controversy surrounding Melissa McLaughlin's diagnosis and the social stigma and internal hierarchy of illness in Emerson Miller's story are evidence of even greater shifts in the trajectory of modern chronic disease. On the one hand, McLaughlin's chronic pain experience rings true to the experiences of millions of patients, particularly women, living with conditions as disparate as migraine/chronic daily headache, irritable bowel syndrome, reflex sympathetic dystrophy (RSD) (also called complex regional pain syndrome, or CRPS) and many other conditions still tinged with the shadow of psychosomatic illness. In her memoir of chronic daily headache and Western attitudes toward pain and gender, Paula Kamen contemplates her "greater privilege to complain," and reflects on her grandparents, who, like most everyone else at the time, were too caught up in survival to focus on maladies such as headaches.[5] For that generation, infectious disease was a greater threat to mortality, and we will see the consequences of that loss of urgency and immediacy in later chapters.

One of the shifts has been in the doctor-patient relationship, which has certainly gone through drastic changes from the "doctor as God" complex of earlier times. Throughout much of the twentieth century it was still common practice for doctors of cancer patients to tell their families their diagnosis, rather than giving the patient the information. We expect more collaboration from our physicians now, and we bring more information to the encounter ourselves. If we have the wherewithal and resources to do so, many of us will shop around and find a better fit rather than settling for a negative relationship with our health care providers.

In his essay "How To Speak Postmodern: Medicine, Illness, and Cultural Change," David B. Morris writes that a distinguishing characteristic of postmodern illness ("postmodern" here refers roughly to the period following World War Two) is that the narrative surrounding illness now often involves the patient.[6] A postmodern view is one that must move beyond the biomedical model of illness that dominated much of the early and mid-twentieth century, a model based on the idea that the body and its ailments can be described in the language of physics and chemistry. That is, disease is something we cure using all the tools at our disposal.[7] This model serves acute illness and injury well, but it falls short for patients who live with ongoing disease.

Given the success in immunization, antibiotic development, and understanding of microbial diseases that characterized the decades following World War Two, this biomedical view of medicine is not surprising. However, with today's technological innovation and the social interaction made possible by Web 2.0, whereby patients are willing to not only swap stories but also experiment with alternative treatment therapies, Morris offers up what he calls a biocultural model as a better fit. Here, illness exists at the "crossroads" of biology and culture, a confusing landscape where all parties involved are increasingly aware of the limits of the rigid biomedical model.[8] This idea of a crossroads is an ever-shifting point at which cultural expectations and assumptions about illness meet scientific inquiry and innovation.

McLaughlin's and Miller's stories are glimpses of this biocultural crossroads. In the former, we see the reservations ascribed to symptoms and conditions that cannot be verified with a blood test or a lab report. In the latter, we see a disease that is easily identified through testing, whose origins we can trace and whose biology is explored in research laboratories and hospitals around the world. Their diagnostic processes are opposites, yet their stories are bound by shared themes and, ultimately, shared experiences.

In tackling these issues, I face challenges of scope and context. Before we can look at the emergence and ongoing adjustments in how we perceive *chronic* disease, we need to establish a basic historical understanding of disease itself. How have scholars, scientists, and physicians thought of the body? What does it mean to be sick? To have a meaningful conversation about the present, we need some context of our past.

Ancient Thinkers with Modern Reach

The Hippocratic oath to "do no harm" takes on added complexity when we factor in the extraordinary means and life-prolonging machines available to us now, but Hippocrates (ca. 460–ca. 377 B.C.) was responsible for more than the pledge so many of us recognize today. He was the first healer in antiquity to move away from the notion that illness and disease were caused by supernatural powers, cosmic forces that could destroy populations at will and who required sacrifices, prayers, and cajoling to spare people. Instead, Hippocrates relied on the power of observation and redefined the role of healer as a true clinician, one who paid close attention to patients' symptoms in order to understand the nature of their diseases. In removing health and illness from the gods and insisting on natural causes and natural cures, Hippocrates caused a profound shift in agency to take place.[9] No longer were patients solely at the mercy of mercurial gods, and no longer were their healers merely present to patch wounds or amputate limbs. This rational, observational medicine centered on the patient, not the disease, and Hippocrates and his followers were interested less in the specifics of singular diseases and more in understanding the natural course of an illness.[10]

The distinction between illness and disease is one that comes up repeatedly in the broader history of chronic illness, with disease being the objective, evidence-based experience of being sick and illness being the subjective, lived experience of patients. In Hippocrates' time, disease was believed to result when an imbalance of the body's natural forces, or humors, occurred. Blood came from the heart and was warm and wet; bile came from the spleen and was black, cold, and dry; phlegm came from the brain and was wet and cold; and lastly, yellow bile, which came from the liver, was warm and dry.[11] While centuries of discovery and understanding would eventually disprove the notion of the four humors, fundamental aspects of Hippocratic medicine still resonate today: diseases manifest differently from individual to individual, and a patient's lifestyle and environment play large roles in determining the course of a disease.[12] The Hippocratics' view was actually quite simple: health represented equilibrium, while illness represented an upset to that harmony.[13]

Influenced by the work of Hippocrates, Plato (ca. 428–ca. 348 B.C.) also believed that a disruption in the body's natural forces—earth, fire, water, and air—caused disease, and that the physician's duty was to advance health by harmonizing body and soul.[14] The mind-body connection and the phrase "sound mind, sound body" that we see and hear often these days, particularly in the growing popularity of complementary and alternative treatments and relaxation techniques, is evident in the Platonic ideal of medicine. As Plato transmitted to us in *The Republic*, Socrates (ca. 470–399 B.C.) viewed health in similar terms, maintaining that virtue, beauty, and spiritual health are mutually dependent, unlike disease, ugliness, and weakness.[15] Like Hippocrates, Plato involved the patient in his treatment of disease—not relying on divine intervention—and also invoked the patient's at least partial responsibility for disease. Platonic healing depended on "the elimination of all evil from body and soul by means of a change in the way of living," whereby the success or failure of treatment also rests with the patient.[16]

Since more of his writing survived than did that of the ancient Greeks, Roman physician Galen (A.D. 129–ca. 199) remains the most prolific ancient writer on medical subjects. He employed the Hippocratic theory to try to understand the nature of disease, and his work with animal cadavers—coupled with his fame and self-promotion—led to misunderstandings of human anatomy that would circulate for a thousand years.[17] Like others of his time, he believed blood was produced in the liver, and his penchant for extreme bloodletting, sometimes until the point of lost consciousness, was derived from the mistaken belief that since women bled monthly and appeared to suffer fewer illnesses than men, bloodletting was an effective way to rid the body of disease. The pulse was another favored topic of inquiry for Galen, but lacking the correct physiological understanding of human anatomy and the circulatory system, his books and writings promoted ideas that would not be disproved until the nineteenth century.[18] The power of his fame and accessibility perpetuated incorrect information about disease, similar to today's landscape in which technology and social media make it possible to widely disperse information and research that may lack accurate or substantive evidence.

While ancient times were characterized by the desire to understand the nature of disease and tie it to physiological imbalances as well as lifestyle, the Middle Ages, influenced by the spread of Christianity, reflected a spiritual understanding of disease and plague as wrought by sin. This is a marked shift from the more naturalistic and rational practice of classical medicine. Early Christian thought emphasized the split between the body and the soul (not the body and the mind), a divine purpose and plan for everything, and the implicit subordination of medicine to religion. Physicians were not healers in the same sense; they tended to the body, while priests were concerned with the more important matters of the soul.[19]

Illness and suffering were viewed as punishment or a test of one's faith, but the early Church also manifested a mission of healing.[20] Since the body was created in the image of God and ultimately belonged to Him, He had the power to heal. The resurrection of Jesus Christ and the glory that waited for the faithful at the Final Judgment were the greatest examples of God's power. The Gospel of Saint Luke, himself a physician, points to several miracles in which the healing power of Christ and his disciples triumphs over bodily disease, including restoring sight to the blind and raising the dead back to life. As Europeans struggled to survive and assimilate the great plagues of the first three centuries of the Christian Era, the notion that "illness is a consequence of sin and not a physical malady to be studied and analyzed as the Greeks did" was rooted in Biblical scripture.[21]

Christianity was just one of many faiths undergoing adaptation as a result of the changing world. It has more emphasis here since some of the themes popular in the Christian response to suffering and disease are still evident today. Even the word *stigma* itself, one so heavily associated with current experiences with disease, has its roots in early Christian tradition. A literal meaning conjures up images of the physical markings of crucifixion, but as psychologist Gregory M. Herek notes, more complex definitions include literal or metaphorical marks that infer an individual is "criminal, villainous, or otherwise deserving of social ostracism, infamy, shame, and condemnation."[22]

Prior to the Black Death in the fourteenth century, it had been eight hundred years since Europe had last been besieged by major epidemics. The collapse of the Roman Empire meant less travel and commerce with Asia and, therefore, less contact with new diseases and infections. Now, with fourteenth-century towns like Venice and Genoa emerging as centers of trade and travel with more distant lands, the opportunity for disease and epidemics to infiltrate a new population was ripe.[23] Increased commerce meant increased urbanization, and poor sanitation and overcrowded conditions meant the population was particularly susceptible to communicable diseases. This relationship between changes in the way people live and work is a constant in the social history of disease.

Bubonic plague, the cause of the Black Death, was thought to infect humans from the fleas carried by rats, though modern experts believe some human-to-human transmission was possible, given how quickly it wreaked havoc. Killing an estimated twenty million people, the Black Death remains Europe's most catastrophic epidemic, having wiped out a quarter of the population.[24] The impact of such devastation on the European psyche is telling. It had become "a crucible of pestilences, spawning the obsessions haunting late medieval imaginations: death, decay, and the Devil . . . the Grim Reaper and the Horsemen of the Apocolypse."[25] Unfortunately, responses to the Black Death are predictable through the lens of history. To the many who believed the plague was the work of divine retribution, acts of self-flagellation, prayer and fasting, and the religious persecution of Jews and others outside the faith were seen as appropriate defenses. Roy Porter recounts the horrific fate of thousands of Jews locked in a wooden building and burned alive, one of many instances of retaliation and violence during the Black Death.[26] Physicians, powerless to effect any substantive treatment for individual patients, could do little to quell the public health debacle unfolding.

French philosopher Michel Foucault's *Panopticism*, published in English translation in 1977, deals graphically with response to plague, describing the total lockdown enforced—the census, the front doors locked and checked by specially appointed officials, the total submission of medical and policy decisions to the magistrates. Order trumps chaos, power dominates disease. Given the rapid transmission and onset of the infection, and the lack of concrete physiological understanding of it, the extreme situation Foucault depicts in seventeenth-century France is understandable, if unappealing. Twenty-first-century movies like *I Am Legend* or *Contagion* tap into similar fears over uncontrollable outbreaks and the fragility of human life in the face of pathogens we cannot fight.

Medieval attitudes toward disease and the body perceived women as the "faulty version" of the male who were weaker because "menstruation and tearfulness displayed a watery, oozing physicality . . . Women were leaky vessels . . . and menstruation was polluting."[27] As patient narrative, research, and history will illustrate, gender remains an incredibly important variable in the chronic illness experience. Partly, this is because more females than males manifest chronic and autoimmune conditions. However, throughout history, deeply ingrained ideas about women as unreliable narrators of their pain and symptoms, as weaker than men, and as histrionic or otherwise "emotional" have had a profound impact on their ability to receive accurate diagnoses and appropriate care.

On the heels of the devastation wrought by the plagues of the Middle Ages, the Renaissance and Enlightenment were periods of progress and advancement. The invention of the printing press and the resulting printed health material made knowledge about the human body and disease (however incomplete) widely available for the first time. The gains in health literacy that printing made possible over time marked a huge shift in the understanding and treatment of diseases.

By the eighteenth century, physicians still couldn't isolate the cause of infectious disease, so Hippocratic thoughts about individual responsibility for illness continued to dominate mindsets. American physician Benjamin Rush emphasized the importance of getting the patient's history directly from the source, and focused on all the daily habits and behaviors that might play a role in the patient's illness. His interest in the association between chronic disease and lifestyle are significant, as is his division between acute and chronic disease.

"In chronic diseases, enquire their complaints far back and the habits of life . . . Pay attention to the phraseology of your patients, for the same ideas are frequently conveyed in different words," Rush counseled his peers.[28] With acute illness, the precise daily habits that took place the week preceding the manifestation of symptoms were particularly important. Rush's emphasis on patient history as a primary diagnostic tool took place in the context of improved standards of living and transportation across Europe and in the United States, which meant a now-predictable rise in diseases associated with indulgence and inactivity. Relying so heavily on patient history and lifestyle was logical, particularly since there was little else physicians could point to in order to assign cause (or blame) for disease.

Other popular theories of the time included a focus on environment and external factors like squalid living conditions and dank areas, though those too brought in associations about wealth, status, and worth. Still, as a precursor to more current attitudes toward patients with chronic disease, this link with lifestyle and behavior is a key concept to carry forward.

The greatest dichotomy of this time period, however, was that while physicians gained new skills and attained a more elevated status, patients themselves saw little benefit from these developments. Even the early use of the microscope shows an interesting lack of focus on the patient, and a divergence from medical research as inherently therapeutic: while physicians used microscopes to study tissue, it wasn't until the nineteenth century's breakthroughs in bacteriology that microscopes were used in the process of treating patients.

Disease in the Nineteenth and Early to Mid-Twentieth Centuries

Simply put, the nineteenth century was the century of the germ. Until physicians could see disease under the microscope, the same kind of guesswork that characterized disease and its treatments from its classical roots persisted. For example, well into the nineteenth century physicians believed that illness came from miasmas—the gases that seeped out from subway systems, garbage dumps, and open graves.[29] The changes wrought by the Industrial Revolution and the emergence of capitalism affected virtually every part of daily life. More people moved to cities and worked in factories, and overall improvements in employment availability and children who could contribute economically to their families meant an increase in population growth. From unsafe working conditions to slums where infectious disease found places to thrive, a now-familiar historical pattern emerged: the technology that yielded improved transportation and innovations in production also paved the way for a new wave of communicable disease and social anxiety.

A fundamental shift in the understanding of disease—and in the way we perceived patients with communicable and other diseases—began with Louis Pasteur's identification of bacteria and the role of germs in causing infection. Before that, leeches, laxatives, and brandy were among the most common cures of the day.[30] By 1881, Pasteur had perfected the vaccination method, though it wouldn't be until 1954 that a polio vaccine suitable and effective for humans was introduced.[31] Nineteenth-century attitudes toward vaccines prevented universal vaccinations from happening. As we will see when we explore current perspectives on vaccines and autism, the combination of fear that the government was encroaching on civil liberties and concern over the safety of the procedures that characterized the opposition to vaccines looms heavily in our twenty-first-century consciousness. The difference between society's perspectives then and now is that in the years between vaccines have largely eliminated many of the most harmful public health risks, such as polio and smallpox.

Vaccination is an approach to disease prevention so profound that it is in large part responsible for the emergence of chronic illness as a domestic public health and social issue in the twentieth century. Enough people did not die or become crippled and incapacitated from infectious disease that they began living long enough to acquire and suffer from chronic conditions. For example, from 1930 to 1980, self-reported illnesses rose by 150 percent, a clear indication that a population that lived longer wasn't necessarily *feeling* better—and an idea that figures prominently in the social history of chronic disease.[32]

Pasteur's work on germ theory ushered in the burgeoning field of microbiology. Using this theory, Pasteur's contemporary Robert Koch was able to identify the bacteria that caused both cholera and tuberculosis (TB).[33] These infections were scourges, particularly in heavily populated urban areas, and brought with them many unfavorable associations and connotations. Perhaps one of the most famous representations of TB appears in Susan Sontag's extended comparison of it to cancer. While cancer was once associated with a repressed personality and middle-class anxiety, TB was the stuff of excess emotion and poverty. In *Illness as Metaphor*, Sontag observed that "TB is a disease of time; it speeds up life, highlights it, spiritualizes it . . . TB is often imagined as a disease of poverty and deprivation—of thin garments, thin bodies, unheated rooms, poor hygiene, inadequate food . . . There was a notion that TB was a wet disease, a disease of humid and dank cities."[34] This process of how identifying the origin of a disease changes the perceptions of patients living with it—or, *fails* to change the perception of patients—is one we still grapple with two centuries later.

In W. Somerset Maugham's revealing early-twentieth-century short story "Sanatorium," assumptions about the "typical" TB patient are powerfully laid bare. In describing one of the patients sent to recover from TB in a sanatorium, the author writes, "He was a stocky, broad-shouldered, wiry little fellow, and the last person you would ever have thought would be attacked by T.B . . . He was a perfectly ordinary man, somewhere between thirty and forty, married, with two children. He lived in a decent suburb. He went up to the City every morning and read the morning paper; he came down from the City every evening and read the evening paper. He had no interests except his business and his family."[35] All the things that make this patient a surprising candidate—he is gainfully employed, stable, married; in short, a respectable man with respectable middle-class tastes and aspirations—are what stand out here. He did not *deserve* his unlikely affliction.

The public health response to disease outbreak in America also reflected the nation's emerging evangelical bent. Since disease was thought to be due to poor hygiene and unsanitary conditions, clean living was not just a health issue but a moral one as well. It fell to religious philanthropists to preach against the sins associated with unclean living, from drinking and immoral behavior to the alleged vices of atheism and greed. Such actions further demarcated the healthy—middle- and upper-class religious activists—from the ill, those languishing in slums whose slovenly living conditions and life choices made them culpable in their sickness. Being able to source the origin of infectious disease to its microbial roots was the first step in breaking down such misconceptions.

Other nineteenth-century developments that influenced the experience of chronic illness today include the advent of anesthesia, the beginning movement toward patient advocacy, and the professionalization of nursing. Until the 1840s, physicians had no effective, safe way to lessen the pain of surgery. The introduction of nitrous oxide, chloroform, and ether produced immense relief from the pain of surgical intervention. It also reflected a shift in physicians' attitudes toward patients and a higher priority on alleviating suffering.

Another advancement in the consideration of the patient can be traced to the nursing profession. Prominent figures like Florence Nightingale and Clara Barton exemplified the holistic approach to patient care that characterizes nursing, and represented a marked departure from the tendency of other medical professionals to focus on singular aspects of a patient's condition (i.e., the cause or the treatment). Galvanized by the suffering of soldiers, Nightingale was stalwart in her work to improve living and sanitary conditions for her patients. The patient as an individual, entitled to respect and compassion, was a concept made flesh by Nightingale and the cadre of professional nurses she mentored. Likewise, activists like Dorothea Dix and Alice Hamilton worked to make public the deplorable living conditions and inhumane treatment of the mentally ill and the urban poor.[36] This indicated a new interest in health-care advocacy, a concept that would wholly redefine the lives of many different types of patients more than a hundred years later, most especially those with chronic diseases.

The world was still in the grip of deadly epidemics, though, as witnessed by the staggering transcontinental death toll of the 1918 influenza pandemic. Updated research suggests that the strain of the influenza virus that sprang up during the 1918–19 flu season killed between thirty and fifty million people globally, and killed an estimated 675,000 Americans. World War One had killed fewer people than the flu pandemic.[37]

Successes in identifying infectious disease and the post–World War Two development of antibiotic therapy led to the assumption that though infections might still cause temporary discomfort, they were no longer a serious threat to either survival or quality of life.[38] Was this a sign of naïveté? Arrogance? Optimism? Or perhaps, a combination of all three? With the benefit of hindsight, the weakness of this position is easy to see: for one, antibiotics only treat certain strains of bacteria, and are not effective in treating the many viruses that still pose a threat to public health. In addition, as we see all too frequently today with infections like methicillin-resistant *Staphylococcus aureus* (MRSA) and flesh-eating *Streptococcus*, bacteria evolve into strains resistant to the medications developed to treat them. As a patient with a compromised immune system who is prone to infections, I know firsthand the danger of antibiotic resistance. As a pre-schooler, I spent several weeks in an isolation room in a hospital, tethered to an IV pole to receive Vancomycin, the drug used to treat staph infections like the one I had spreading from my ears to my brain. Knowing that some staph infections are now resistant to Vancomycin, a powerful "end-of-the-line" treatment for these life-threatening infections, scares me. Similarly, with only a few antibiotic options left that reliably treat my lung infections, resistance is not just a buzz-worthy topic for me; it is a real concern.

For better and worse, twentieth-century experiences with diseases like polio forever altered the way we view medical science's ability to treat disease. At last, humanity could respond to the infectious epidemics that had wreaked havoc for centuries and do more than merely identify them—we could actually *prevent* them. Outside the spheres of public health and research, we don't hear or talk too much about polio anymore; its omission in our lexicon is a luxury modern medicine affords us. But for the generation forced to dwell in iron lungs and the legions permanently crippled by polio, its specter was menacing. Many of the illnesses we grapple with today are a product of the way we live and work, just as living and working conditions in the past contributed to the rise of polio. Roy Porter deftly characterized the complex relationship between human progress and disease when he wrote, "Thus to many, from classical poets up to the prophets of modernity, disease has seemed the dark side of development, its Jekyll-and-Hyde double; progress brings pestilences, society sickness."[39]

Though ancient in origin, the emergence of polio as a major medical threat in the 1900s can be traced directly to the processes of urbanization. Spread through infected fecal matter, the dominant strains of the polio virus were introduced early on to infants who dwelled in crowded homes with rudimentary plumbing, sanitation, and hygiene. Once more modern forms of sanitation and waste removal and treatment were developed in the 1900s, the immunity that early exposure to the virus gave patients happened less frequently.[40] As immunity decreased, incidence of the more serious manifestation of polio, paraltyic polio, which involved the nervous system, increased. By the 1950s, polio kicked up most severely during the warm summer months and primarily affected children. Parents fled urban areas and communities banned the use of public swimming pools.[41] The year 1952 brought with it the worst polio epidemic in American history; 58,000 cases were reported, including 3,145 deaths.[42]

That same year, 1952, Jonas Salk tested the first polio vaccine. He used a dead virus injected into patients to help build up natural immunity, and in 1954 more than one million children were given test vaccinations.[43] Since polio was a disease that primarily affected children, treating it was a cause particularly vaunted by the American public. Children are understandably at the top of the illness hierarchy. By the late 1950s, a live virus was used to produce an oral vaccine, which was more popular since it meant patients didn't need any shots. The World Health Organization (WHO) made fully eradicating polio a worldwide effort in 1985.[44]

Industrialization and urbanization were responsible for the emergence of diseases like polio, but changes in the way people communicated were responsible for spreading public health goals, too. Disease wasn't just about scientific theories; it was a social phenomenon. The America that emerged after World War Two was fighting a war in Korea and was consumed with the Cold War and McCarthyism, and a new form of technology brought these events—and, more importantly, the intellectual and emotional basis for them—into the home. Television was an important player in spreading the "gospel of health" and promoting newly focused public health and medical research goals. A well-run state depended on people adopting a preferred public health agenda, and mass communication of health literature allowed that to happen.[45] Putting health information in the hands of the general public took it out of the exclusive domain of the doctor in the laboratory or operating room and brought it into the realm of the patient's narrative and subjective experience.

It is in this context that we reconsider Melissa McLaughlin's chronic fatigue syndrome and fibromyalgia, or Emerson Miller's HIV, the latest additions to an increasingly widening scope of conditions we can treat but we cannot cure.

"The fact that you're just not going to get better seems unbelievable to most people, I guess," says Melissa McLaughlin. One frustration for her is people who can't understand that patients cannot control or fix everything. "It's easier for them to believe that there is something you can control . . . There must be something you can do that you aren't doing! Eating raw foods, forcing yourself to exercise, thinking your way out of it, trying the latest drugs that promise a cure in their commercial: something should work, and if you're not better, then you're not working hard enough. It's frustrating, it's everywhere (even, sometimes, in my own mind), and it's just wrong. It's just wrong: I can't think or eat or exercise my way out of these illnesses, no matter how hard I try." Even Melissa's doctors followed suit, urging her to exercise more often even though it made her pain and fatigue much worse.

On the other hand, we have our great fear of HIV, the infectious disease that does not bend to our will. Shame is often embedded in its mode of transmission, and so far its wily ability to mutate has made it impervious to the very same vaccination process that revolutionized modern medical science. Emerson Miller doesn't believe he will see a cure in the lifetime of current researchers, and, in fact, he worries that the progress we have made may actually have a negative impact on the search for a cure and on vigilance against the spread of HIV.

"I don't want the sense of urgency to go away," he says, hoping that the knowledge there is a drug cocktail that can effectively reduce viral load does not mean people will take the disease less seriously, particularly those who may contract the virus through preventable life choices.

The journey from Plato and Socrates to the Enlightenment and Industrialization to more modern public health advances is a circuitous one. By the middle of the twentieth century, the ability of scientists, physicians, and public health officials to alter the course of diseases that once devastated the population made it possible for people to adapt their thoughts on illness and disability; no longer were they considered to be inevitable and immovable components of daily life. This attitude would have strong re-percussions for the next generation of patients, the ones touched by the other big medical emergence of the postmodern era: chronic illness. The period immediately after World War Two was a time of what scholar Gerald Grob describes as irresistible progress, a time when it seemed like science was on the brink of curing so much of what ailed us.[46] With so many concrete victories to point to, the existence of illnesses that would not go away—chronic conditions that were somehow beyond the reach of medical science—would appear that much more unpalatable.

CHAPTER 2

An Awakening
Medicine and Illness in
Post–World War Two America

E V E R Y semester, when I ask my health sciences students to define what medical ethics means to them, I usually hear the same chorus of responses: treating the patient as a whole person. Advocating for the patient. My nursing students often chime in with the term "non-malfeasance"— avoiding doing harm to the patient. They often share examples of when those ethics were challenged without divulging personal details, since patient confidentiality is taken seriously in our classroom, thanks to the Health Insurance Portability and Accountability Act (HIPAA) of 1996. Teenage patients who want a course of treatment different from what their parents want for them, or an elderly patient's wishes not being respected by the next of kin tasked with difficult decisions, are common examples. Usually, it is when we explore instances of perceived lapses in judgment or ethics that we circle around to the most exhaustive understanding of why the students choose to define ethics as they do.

Perched over Boston's bustling Huntington Avenue in our fourth-floor classroom at Northeastern University, steps from Harvard teaching hospitals like Brigham and Women's and Beth Israel Deaconess Medical Center, as well as other renowned institutions like Children's Hospital, the Dana-Farber Cancer Institute, and the Joslin Diabetes Clinic, we are all fortunate. When I need to, I can take a left down Huntington Avenue, walking past the take-out restaurants and dive bars with dollar wing specials, past where the E Line street-level trolley cuts through the main thoroughfare, filled with high school students, nurses and medical residents, young mothers with children in strollers, and college students with iPod ear buds. When I walk through Brigham's main revolving door I am no longer a writer and health sciences writing lecturer; I am a patient with a rare disease who depends on the innovative treatments and technology at hospitals like this. Quite literally, I am crossing Sontag's threshold from the kingdom of the well into the kingdom of the sick. In many respects, I know this kingdom and its attendant customs and interactions more intimately than I do the realm of the healthy. Appointments and hospital admissions are frequent in my world, and the diagnostic tests, procedures, and treatments I sign consent forms for are a routine part of my life.

My students often make this same walk down Huntington to their respective clinical and co-op placements, field placements the school arranges, minutes from their dorms and apartments and their classrooms and labs. They learn about patient care in some of the most medically advanced and prestigious research hospitals in the world. They too cross into another kingdom, shedding their college student personas and adopting the mindset of the health care apprentice. We each have our roles, and it is easy to forget that not all patients and providers have access like this.

My students' definitions of medical ethics are on point, but it isn't without more probing and more discussion that we land upon the topics of informed consent and patients' rights. I think this is partially a good thing; they see these principles at work so regularly in their rotations that the principles are just that: routine. Lists of patients' rights are posted on hospital walls and in emergency room bays throughout hospitals. Informed consent for procedures big and small often—not always, but often enough—entails a quick overview and a dash of a perfunctory signature. But every now and then, a student will question what we often take at face value.

How informed is consent if, say, the patient doesn't have a good grasp of English and there isn't time for a translator, or the resources to provide one? To what extent do patients who have no health insurance and therefore limited ability to seek different care have their basic rights upheld?

How helpful or equitable are online resources if they assume a digital literacy and access that some patients don't have?

Most often, it is when something goes wrong that we stop and think about the potential risks listed on the procedures we agree to undergo, or consider just what it means to be treated with respect and dignity regardless of our origin, religion, or financial status. Because those of us with appropriate access to consent forms and patients' rights have the luxury to navigate a medical establishment that is at least moderately successful in upholding these basic promises, we don't have to stop and consider them as much as we might otherwise.

The ethical treatment of patients may depend in part on whether we think our illnesses say more about us than our health. On the surface, if we are just looking at obesity rates, cardiovascular disease, or a decline in physical activity precipitated by a digital lifestyle, it is easy to claim that yes, perhaps they do. If we consider the association between the environment in which we live and the risk of developing certain cancers and other conditions, then that is another layer of probability. However, the question probes at something much deeper than that. If our illnesses reveal strength or weakness in us, then so too does the way we treat the individual patient living with illness.

In the decades just following World War Two and leading up to the social justice movements of the 1960s and '70s, many of the concepts most of us take for granted had a fairly egregious track record. Informed consent was at best an afterthought, at worst deliberately ignored, and medical decision making was too often deeply skewed toward those with power. The 1950s and '60s were a pivotal turning point in patients' rights, ethics, and medical decision making. For patients living with chronic and degenerative diseases, the timing of this was critical.

Chronic Illness as an Emerging Priority

On the heels of World War Two, America was coming down from the heady throes of patriotism and was exposed to more innovative medical technology. The establishment of the independent, nonprofit national Commission on Chronic Illness in May 1949[1] indicated a growing awareness of the demands of chronic disease. The Commission on Chronic Illness was a joint creation of the American Hospital Association, the American Medical Association, and the American Public Welfare Association[2] and its initial goals included gathering and sharing information on how to deal with the "many-sided problem" of chronic illness; undertaking new studies to help address chronic illness; and formulating local, state, and federal plans for dealing with chronic illness.[3] This included plans to dispel society's belief that chronic illness was a hopeless scenario, create programs that would help patients reclaim a productive space in society, and coordinate disease-specific groups with a more universal program that would more effectively meet the needs of all patients with chronic illness, regardless of diagnosis.[4]

These goals indicate that when chronic illness was emerging as a necessary part of the postwar medical lexicon, it was seen as a social issue, not just a physical or semantic one. Many of these goals are the same ones patients and public health officials point to today, signaling that either the commission was particularly forward-thinking—or, that we have yet to mobilize and systematically address the unique needs of the chronically ill the way other movements have mobilized in the past.

Still, the Commission on Chronic Illness was an important concrete step in the process to recognize and address chronic illness. It defined chronic illness as any impairment characterized by at least one of the following: permanence, residual disability, originating in irreversible pathological alteration, or requiring extended care or supervision.[5] Now, we have many variations of the same theme. Sometimes, the length of time symptoms must persist differs; sometimes, the focus is on ongoing treatment rather than supervision. Rosalind Joffe, a patient with chronic illness who is a life coach specializing in helping executives with chronic illness stay employed, offers three important characteristics experts agree are often found in chronic illness: the symptoms are invisible, symptoms and disease progression vary from person to person, and the disease progression and worsening or improvement of symptoms are impossible to predict.[6] I've always found the "treatable, not curable" mantra a helpful one in discussing chronic illness, since it allows for all those variances in diagnoses, disease course, and outcomes. In some cases, treatment could be as simple as an anti-inflammatory drug to manage mild arthritis or daily thyroid medication to correct an imbalanced thyroid hormone level. At the other end of the spectrum are diseases like cystic fibrosis, where the treatment progresses to include organ transplantation (which is a life-extender, not a cure).

To get a sense of just how broad the spectrum of what we could define as chronic illness is, consider sinusitis, a very common chronic condition affecting some thirty-one million patients annually.[7] Its frequency, duration, and treatment (because even those who undergo surgery for it are rarely fully cured) technically fit the basic meaning of a chronic illness, a prime example of the utility of substituting "condition" for "illness." However, sinus congestion is not the ailment we usually associate with chronically ill patients. That this umbrella term reaches far enough to encompass AIDS is a telling shift and adds to that basic premise that chronic illness is treatable, not curable.

More than being a straightforward counterpart of acute illness, the very notion of chronic illness is one rooted in social and class consciousness. Ours is a society that values youth, physical fitness, and overachievement. By the middle of the twentieth century, this elevation of the importance of the perceptions of others played out in rigid social conformity, as well as in anxiety about that conformity. Scholars and writers of the time worried that people were living in "slavish compliance to the opinions of others— neighbors, bosses, the corporation, the peer group, the anonymous public."[8] Given the external events of the time—McCarthyism, the Cold War, the space race—it is not hard to see why maintaining the status quo and the cloak of homogeneity would have been appealing to many, and why in the ensuing years, so many would rebel from that same conformity.

As I write this, the term "self-improvement" conjures up images of extreme dieting and aggressive cosmetic surgeries and enhancements more often than it does industriousness or work ethic. In fact, the drive for perfection often spurs the desire for short cuts or immediate results our

technology-driven culture makes possible. If science can improve on im-
perfections, shouldn't we take advantage of its largesse? The middle of the
twentieth century ushered in the idea that we must somehow stack up
across all social and professional strata in our lives. News headlines are
filled with stories that track stars' adventures in surgical reconstruction,
and daytime television commercials are rife with weight loss ads and
other enhancement products that offer big rewards with supposedly little
risk. This upsurge in enhancement technologies is what physician, philosopher, and bioethicist Carl Elliott calls the American obsession with fitting
in, countered by the American anxiety over fitting in too well. The very
nature of chronic illness—debilitating symptoms, physical side effects of
medications, the gradual slowing down as diseases progress—is antithetical to the cult of improvement and enhancement that so permeates pop
culture.

Autoimmune diseases, which affect nearly twenty-four million Americans,[9] are a prime example of chronic illnesses that defy self-improvement.
At their core, autoimmune disorders occur when the body mistakenly
begins to attack itself. The concept first took root in 1957, but in *The Autoimmune Epidemic*, Donna Jackson Nakazawa points out that it wasn't until
the 1970s that the concept gained widespread acceptance. While heart
disease, cancer, and other chronic conditions had been tracked for decades, as late as the 1990s no government or disease-centered organization
had collected data on how many Americans lived with the often baffling
conditions that make up autoimmune diseases.[10] The mid-twentieth-century
America in which the notion of autoimmune disease made its debut represents a pivotal time period in the evolution of chronic illness. The country
had just moved past the frenetic pace of immunization and research that
followed World War Two. Patients' rights and informed consent began to
be recognized as important issues, particularly with the emerging field of
organ transplantation, and those topics plus the advent of managed care
plans in the 1960s each contributed to the beginning of a marked change
in how medicine and society looked at disease.

With autoimmune diseases, the specific part of the body that is attacked manifests itself in a wide variety of conditions, from the joints and

muscles (rheumatoid arthritis and lupus) to the myelin sheath in the central nervous system (multiple sclerosis) to the colon or muscles (Crohn's and polymyositis). It isn't so much a question of whether autoimmune disorders are "new" conditions as it is a question of correctly identifying them and sourcing the origin of that fateful trigger. Sometimes, something as innocuous as a common, low-grade virus can be the trigger that jumpstarts the faulty immune response, and research suggests many of us carry genes that leave us more predisposed to developing autoimmune disease. However, when we look at alarming increases in the number of patients being diagnosed with conditions like lupus, the role of the environment, in particular the chemicals that go into the household products we use, the food we consume, and the technology we employ every day, is of increasing significance.

Nakazawa takes a strong position on this relationship: "During the four or five decades that science lingered at the sidelines . . . another cultural drama was unfolding in America, the portentous ramifications of which were also slipping under the nation's radar. Throughout the exact same decades science was dismissing autoimmunity, the wheels of big industry were moving into high gear across the American landscape, augmenting the greatest industrial growth spurt of all time."[11]

It is simply not possible to discuss disease in purely scientific language. Culture informs the experience of illness, and living with illness ultimately shapes culture. From the interconnectedness of the way we work and communicate virtually to the way we eat to the products we buy, the innovation that has so drastically changed the course of daily life and culture has an unquestionable impact on health and on the emergence of disease. Technology and science inform culture as well, and cultural mores influence what research we fund, and how we use technology.

If we look at current perspectives and definitions of chronic illness from the Centers for Disease Control and Prevention (CDC), there is a telling change in focus from earlier iterations. In detailing the causes of chronic disease, which current data suggest almost one out of every two Americans lives with, the CDC listed lack of physical activity, poor nutrition, tobacco use, and alcohol consumption as responsible for much of the illness, suffering, and premature death attributed to chronic diseases in 2010.[12] Given that heart disease, stroke, and cancer account for more than 50 percent of deaths annually, and each is linked to lifestyle and behaviors, it is not a surprise that these four factors are highlighted.[13] Such emphasis implies something more than merely causation. It denotes agency on the part of patients whose choices and behaviors are at least somewhat complicit in their illnesses. This parallels older attitudes toward infectious diseases: if patients weren't living a certain way (in squalor) or acting a certain way (lasciviously), they wouldn't be sick. At the same time, it separates certain chronic conditions and the patients who live with them from the forward momentum of medical science: we can kill bacteria, we can eradicate diseases through vaccination, we can transplant organs, but the treatment and prevention of many conditions is the responsibility of the patient.

Questions of correlation and causation depend on data. It was during the post–World War Two time period that the methodical collection of statistics on chronic disease began. In the America President Dwight D. Eisenhower inherited in the 1950s, the average lifespan was sixty-nine years. Huge trials were under way to develop a new polio vaccine and new treatments for polio, and heart disease and stroke were more widely recognized as the leading causes of death from noninfectious disease. In 1956, Eisenhower signed the National Health Survey Act, authorizing a continuing survey to gather and maintain accurate statistical information on the type, incidence, and effects of illness and disability in the American population. The resulting National Health Interview Survey (1957) and the National Health Examination Survey (1960) produced data that helped researchers identify and understand risk factors for common chronic diseases like cardiovascular disease and cancer.[14] These developments, which occurred right before the Surgeon General's seminal 1964 report on smoking and lung cancer, revealed an awareness of the pattern between how we lived and the diseases that affected us the most.

The legacy of this association between smoking (a behavior) and lung cancer (an often preventable disease) and policies to reduce smoking in the United States has helped shape public health in the twentieth and twenty-first centuries. From seat belt laws to smoke-free public spaces, the idea that government could at least partially intervene in personal decision making and safety issues started to gain real traction in mid-twentieth-century America. An aggressive (and successful) public health campaign to vaccinate against infectious diseases like polio was one thing; moving from infectious, indiscriminate disease to individual choice and behavior was quite another, and backlash against such public health interventions was strident.

Dr. Barry Popkin, a professor in the Department of Nutrition at the University of North Carolina, is on the front lines of the political debate over taxing soda and other sugary beverages and sees similarities in the pushback against policies like the beverage tax. He points to the public health success in saving lives through seat belt laws, or to data showing that the taxing of cigarettes cuts smoking and saves thousands of lives. "It's the same with fluoridizing water," he notes, adding how in the 1950s the American Medical Association accused President Eisenhower of participating in a Communist plot to poison America's drinking water. "There's not a single public health initiative that hasn't faced these arguments," he says.

At the same time these data collection and public health programs took off, the National Institutes of Health (NIH), a now-familiar and influential research organization, gained prominence. Originally formed in 1930, it wasn't until 1946 that the NIH took on the kind of power that we recognize today. The medical research boon ushered in by World War Two and bolstered by the Committee on Medical Research (CMR) threatened to retreat to prewar levels, a move that politicians and scientists alike were loath to see happen. They rallied to increase funding and support of the NIH. Tapping into the patriotic fervor of the time, they argued that medicine was on the cusp of its greatest achievements, from antibiotics to chemotherapy, and that supporting continued research wasn't just for the well-being of Americans as individuals but was critical to national self-interest, too.[15] The timing of the combination of increased technology and patriotic zeal undoubtedly benefited researchers, and in many ways it benefited patients, too. However, the case for national self-interest also created a serious gap when it came to individual patients' rights.

Not surprisingly, military metaphors were often invoked to champion the cause: the battle against disease was in full effect. War, long considered "good" for medicine, was also the physical catalyst for the increased focus on medical research and innovations. Military language first came into favor in the late 1800s, when bacteria and their biological processes were identified, and it continued to proliferate as researchers began to understand more and more about how diseases worked. By the early 1970s, the application of military terms to the disease process was troubling enough to attract the precision lens of essayist Susan Sontag's prose. She wrote, "Cancer cells do not simply multiply; they are 'invasive.' Cancer cells 'colonize' from the original tumor to far sites in the body, first setting up tiny outposts . . . Treatment also has a military flavor. Radiotherapy uses the metaphors of aerial warfare; patients are 'bombarded' with toxic rays. And chemotherapy is chemical warfare, using poisons."[16] The problem is, this scenario leaves little room for those who fight just as hard and do not win.

It is no coincidence that the tenor of the National Cancer Act of 1971, signed into law in December of that year by President Richard M. Nixon, reflected this military attitude. The act, characterized as "bold legislation that mobilized the country's resources to fight cancer," aimed to accelerate research through funding.[17] Just as experts and politicians were unabashedly enthusiastic that infectious disease would soon be conquered with the new tools at their disposal, those involved in cancer treatment believed we were on the precipice of winning this particular "war," too. On both fronts, this success-at-all-costs attitude would have profound implications for patients with chronic illness.

Patient Rights, Provider Privilege:
Medical Ethics in the 1950s–1970s

Until the mid-1960s, decisions about care and treatment fell under the domain of the individual physician, even if those decisions involved major ethical and social issues.[18] Whether it was navigating who should receive then groundbreaking kidney transplants or what constituted quality of life when it came to end-of-life decision making, these pivotal moments of conflict in modern-day patients' rights and informed consent took the sacrosanct doctor-patient relationship and transformed it into something larger than itself.

A major call for ethical change came in the form of a blistering report from within the medical establishment itself. In 1966, anesthesiologist and researcher Henry K. Beecher published his famous whistle-blowing article in the *New England Journal of Medicine* that detailed numerous abuses of patients' rights and patients' dignity. In doing so, he brought to light the sordid underside of the rigorous clinical trials pushed forth under the guise of patriotism in the 1940s. The examples that constituted Beecher's list of dishonor included giving live hepatitis viruses to retarded patients in state institutions to study their etiology, and injecting live cancer cells into elderly and senile patients without disclosing the cells were cancerous to see how their immune systems responded.[19] Such abuses were all too common in post–World War Two medical research, which social medicine historian David Rothman accurately describes as having "lost its intimate directly therapeutic character."[20] Is the point of research to advance science or to improve the life of the patient? The two are not mutually inclusive. The loss Rothman describes cannot be glossed over, and the therapeutic value of treatments and approaches is something we continue to debate today. So significant was this disclosure of abuse that Beecher was propelled to the muckraker ranks of environmentalist Rachel Carson (author of *Silent Spring*), antislavery icon Harriet Beecher Stowe (author of *Uncle Tom's Cabin*, and not a relative of Henry Beecher), and food safety lightning rod Upton Sinclair (author of *The Jungle*). In the tradition of these literary greats, Beecher's article brought to light an indictment of research ethics so great that it transformed medical decision making.[21]

While war might have been good for medicine in terms of expediency and efficiency, it was often catastrophic for the subjects of the clinical trials it spurred. The Nuremberg Code (1947) was the first international document to guide research ethics. It was a formal response to the horrific human experiments, torture, and mass murder perpetrated by Nazi doctors during World War Two. It paved the way for voluntary consent, meaning subjects can consent to participate in a trial, can consent without force or coercion, and that the risks and benefits involved in clinical trials are explained to them in a comprehensive manner. Building on this, the Declaration of Helsinki (1964) was the World Medical Association's attempt to emphasize the difference between care that provides direct benefit for the patient and research that may or may not offer direct benefit.[22]

More than any other document, the Patient's Bill of Rights, officially adopted by the American Hospital Association in 1973, reflected the changing societal attitudes toward the doctor-patient relationship and appropriate standards of practice. Though broad concepts included respectful and compassionate care, the specifics of the document emphasized the patient's right to privacy and the importance of clarity in explaining facts necessary for informed consent. Patient activists were critical of the inability to enforce these provisions or mete out penalties, and they found the exception that allowed a doctor to withhold the truth about health status when the facts might harm the patient to be both self-serving and disingenuous. Still, disclosure of diagnosis and prognosis is truly a modern phenomenon. Remember that in the early 1960s, almost all physicians didn't tell their patients when they had cancer; in one study, a staggering 90 *percent* of physicians called this standard practice. As a testament to these wide-scale changes, by the late 1970s most physicians shared their findings with their patients.[23]

Certainly the lingering shadow of the infamous Tuskegee syphilis study reflects the ongoing question of reasonable informed consent. In the most well-known ethical failure in twentieth-century medicine, researchers in the Tuskegee experiment knowingly withheld treatment from hundreds of poor blacks in Macon County, Alabama, many of whom had syphilis and were never told this, so that the researchers could see how the disease progressed. Informed consent was not present, since crucial facts of the experiment were deliberately kept from the men, who were also largely illiterate. The experiment began in 1932, and researchers from the U.S. Public Health Service told the men they were getting treatment for "bad blood." In exchange for participation, the men were given free medical exams and free meals. Even after a standard course of treatment using penicillin was in place for syphilis in 1947, the appropriate treatment was kept from the subjects. In short, researchers waited and watched the men die from a treatable disease so they could use the autopsies to better understand the disease process.[24]

The experiment lasted an intolerable forty years, until an Associated Press news article broke the story on July 25, 1972. Reporter Jean Heller wrote, "For 40 years, the U.S. Public Health Service has conducted a study in which human guinea pigs, not given proper treatment, have died of syphilis and its side effects." In response, an ad hoc advisory panel was formed at the behest of the Assistant Secretary for Health and Scientific Affairs. It found the experiment "ethically unjustified," meaning that whatever meager knowledge was gained paled in comparison to the enormous (often lethal) risks borne by the subjects, and in October 1972, the panel advised the study be stopped. It did finally stop one month later, and by 1973, a class action lawsuit was filed on behalf of the men and their families. The settlement, reached in 1974, awarded $10 million and lifetime medical care for participants and, later, for their wives, widows, and children.[25] A formal apology for the egregious abuse of power and disrespect for human dignity did not come until President Bill Clinton apologized on behalf of the country in 1997. "What was done cannot be undone," he said. "But we can end the silence. We can stop turning our heads away. We can look at you in the eye and finally say, on behalf of the American people: what the United States government did was shameful."[26]

The lack of informed consent was a major aspect of the morally and ethically unjustified Tuskegee experiment. Similarly, it is hard to argue that orphans, prisoners, and other populations that had served as recruiting grounds for experiments throughout the late nineteenth century and much of the twentieth century could have freely objected to or agreed to participate in experiments—freedom of choice being a hallmark of supposed "voluntary participation." Widespread coercion undoubtedly took place. The rush to develop vaccinations and more effective treatments for diseases during World War Two blurred the line between medical care that was patient-centered and experimentation that fell short of this criterion. It is tempting to think such distasteful subject matter is in the past, but considering how many millions of patients with chronic illness depend on and participate in research trials to improve and perhaps even save their lives, it is an undeniable part of the present, too. When we factor in the complex issue of informed consent and the use of DNA in clinical trials today, we can start to see just how thorny these ethical questions remain.

Another poignant example of a breach in medical ethics is revealed by author Rebecca Skloot in *The Immortal Life of Henrietta Lacks*. The riveting narrative traces the cells taken from a poor black mother who died of cervical cancer in 1951. Samples of her tumor were taken without her knowledge. Unlike other human cells that researchers attempted to keep alive in culture, Henrietta's cells (called HeLa for short) thrived and reproduced a new generation every twenty-four hours. Billions of HeLa cells now live in laboratories around the world, have been used to develop drugs for numerous conditions, and have aided in the understanding of many more. So prolific are the cells and their research results that some people consider them one of the most important medical developments of the past hundred years.[27] And yet despite the enormity and immortality of Henrietta Lacks's cells and the unquestionable profits their experiments have yielded, scientists had no consent to use them, and her descendants were never given the chance to benefit from them.

On the heels of Henry K. Beecher's whistle-blowing article and heated debate over transplantation and end-of-life care, U.S. senators Edward Kennedy and Walter Mondale spearheaded Congress's creation of a national commission on medical ethics in 1973. This helped solidify a commitment to collective (rather than individual) decision making and cemented the emergence of bioethics as a distinct field.[28] With advances in reproductive technology, stem-cell research, and other boundary-pushing developments in medicine we see today, the importance of bioethics is far-reaching. New rules were put into place for researchers working with human subjects to prevent a "self-serving calculus of risks and benefits," and written documentation came to replace word-of-mouth orders. Now, the ubiquitous medical chart that had once been a private form of communication primarily for physicians was a public document that formally recorded conversations between patients and physicians. In 1974, Congress signed into law the National Research Act, which created the National Commission for the Protection of Human Subjects of Biomedical and Behavioral Research. This commission was tasked with identifying the principles that should govern experiments involving human subjects and then suggesting ways to improve protection of participants.[29]

Physicians were divided about the various changes and interventions from politicians, public policy experts, ethicists, and legal experts that emerged during this time period. While some of the most powerful disclosures (such as the Beecher article) came from physicians themselves, many also feared the intrusion into the private relationship between doctor and patient and the resulting changes in power they made possible. When physicians at the Peter Bent Brigham Hospital (now Brigham and Women's Hospital) in Boston successfully transplanted a kidney from one identical twin to another in 1954, it was a milestone in surgical history as well as in collective decision making. Previously, in the closed relationship between physician and patient, the treating physician was responsible for exhausting every means of treatment for that patient. Quite simply, this model did not give physicians the answers for the complex new set of problems that arose once kidney transplants moved from the experimental to the therapeutic stage. Was it ethical, some wondered, to remove a healthy organ from a healthy donor, a procedure that could be considered "purposeful infliction of harm?"[30] Even with donor consent, was participation truly voluntary, particularly when family members were asked to donate? How should physicians handle the triage and allocation of such a scarce resource? These questions were too complicated for the individual physician to address.

Kidney transplantation, which was soon followed by advances in heart transplantation, raised yet another crucial ethical question for physicians, patients, and society at large: How should we define death, especially when one patient's death could potentially benefit another patient? For those languishing with end-stage illness and chronic disease, as well as the huge number of patients who would go on to receive transplants in coming decades, there was hardly a more important question. As transplantation increased, it became clear that using heart death as the definition would not work, since heart death put other transplantable organs at risk.

However, transplants weren't the only impetus for a new definition: the process of dying itself was undergoing enormous change. Part of this change began from within the physical hospital itself. Intensive care units became more standard in hospitals beginning in the 1950s, and the advanced life-supporting equipment they made use of meant that more people died in the hospital than in their bedrooms. By the 1960s, 75 percent of those who were dying were in a hospital or nursing home for at least eight days prior to death. As critic Jill Lepore wrote in the *New Yorker* in 2009, "For decades now, life expectancy has been rising. But the longer we live the longer we die."[31] In 2009, the median length of time patients spent in hospice—palliative services for those facing terminal illness—prior to death was 21.1 days. This figure includes hospice patients who died in hospitals, nursing homes, rehabilitation centers, and private residences.[32] This physical shift in space paralleled an intellectual and moral shift in attitudes toward death and, inevitably, toward disease. Both now involved and were practically indistinguishable from the institution of medicine and all the machines, interventions, and expectations that entailed.

This also meant that while respirators may have kept many patients alive in that their hearts were beating, the substance and quality of that life and the vitality of their brain function was questionable. No case exemplified this struggle more than that of Karen Ann Quinlan—a case that became every bit as important for medical ethics and end-of-life decisions as the revelations about the Tuskegee experiment had been for informed consent and ethical research. The twenty-one-year-old Quinlan mixed drugs and too much alcohol one night in 1975, and friends found her not breathing; her oxygen-deprived brain sustained significant damage, and she was left in a persistent vegetative state with a respirator controlling her breathing. When it was clear to her parents there was no room for improvement, they asked her physicians to remove her respirator. They refused, saying she did not meet the criteria for brain death. Remember that practical applications of the definition of brain death were primarily for the emerging field of transplantation, not for issues related to quality of life and prolonging life. In the same way physicians didn't have a viable frame-work for the ethics of organ allocation on their own, this conceptual frame-work offered little guidance to the Quinlans. Next, the state of New Jersey asserted that it would prosecute any physicians who helped the young woman die. Joseph Quinlan, Karen Ann's father, took his request to court and was first denied; eventually, the New Jersey Supreme Court ruled in his favor, noting that her death would be from natural causes and therefore could not be considered a homicide.[33]

Though some low-level basic brain function remained, all Karen Ann's cognitive and emotional capabilities were wiped out. Lepore reports that pressed to testify as to her mental abilities, one medical expert charac-terized the extent of her injuries in the following manner: "The best way I can describe this would be to take the situation of an anencephalic mon-ster. An anencephalic monster is an infant that's born with no cerebral hemisphere . . . If you take a child like this, in the dark, and you put a flash-light in back of the head, the light comes out of the pupils. They have no brain. O.K.?"[34]

No, there was certainly no road map for scenarios like this in 1975, and the Quinlan case brought the bedside discussion of death to the gov-ernment. It would take Karen Ann Quinlan ten long years to die from in-fection, but by that point the legal and ethical quagmire consumed those inside and outside the medical community. Similar to the way the right to life would grip those of us who watched the Terri Schiavo case and the fight her parents waged to keep her feeding tube inserted unfold in 2005, the Quinlan case was emotionally fraught and captured the attention of many, even those on the outside. The difference between the two cases— one of which is cast as the right to die, while the other represents the fight for the right to life—is, of course, historical and social context.

In 1968, Pope Paul VI issued the influential encyclical letter entitled "Of Human Life," which argued for the sanctity of life beginning at the moment of conception, a central argument used by pro-life factions. In 1973, the United States Supreme Court ruled in *Roe v. Wade*, further po-larizing both sides of the abortion rights debate. Add to this the growing fascination with the institutionalized nature of dying and the not-too-distant shadow of Nazi atrocities, and the fray the Quinlans joined that fateful day in 1975 was rife with agendas, perspectives, and controversy surrounding death. The Quinlan case embodied all these competing forces and beliefs, and its legacy continues in conversations about how to die today. We are still fascinated with death, though the focus now is on the role of government in end-of-life decisions. The kerfuffle over alleged "death panels" that health care reform precipitated in 2010 illustrates this anxiety over who is involved in dying all too well.

The Advent of Medicare

Because experimentation and exploitation so often involved minorities, the burgeoning movement to reform medical experimentation on humans was closely linked with the various civil rights movement of the 1960s and '70s. Decisions about experimentation were no longer seen as the province solely of physicians, nor were the attendant issues strictly medical ones. Now, they were open to political, academic, legal, and philosophical debates. At the same time legislation was enacted to better protect human subjects, another groundbreaking development for patients (and for the role of government in shaping health care policy) took shape: Medicare. According to the Centers for Medicare and Medicaid Services, President Franklin D. Roosevelt felt that health insurance was too controversial to try to include in his Social Security Act of 1935, which provided unemployment benefits, old-age insurance, and maternal-child health.[35] It wasn't until 1965 that President Lyndon B. Johnson got Medicare and Medicaid enacted as part of the Social Security Amendments, extending health coverage to almost all Americans over the age of sixty-five and, in the case of Medicaid, providing health services to those who relied on welfare payments.[36]

In 1972, President Nixon expanded Medicare to include Americans under sixty-five who received Social Security Disability Insurance (SSDI) payments as well as individuals with end-stage renal disease. The way Medicare was set up was not an accurate reflection of the chronic conditions many of its recipients had. At its inception in 1966, its coverage, benefits, and criteria for determining the all-important medical necessity were all directed to the treatment of acute, episodic illness. This model, along with increased payment rates for physicians who treated Medicare patients, would continue virtually unchecked or unchanged for twenty-five years.[37] It reflects the biomedical approach to disease, one that emphasizes treatments and cures, but it falls apart when it comes to patients with chronic disease, who make up the majority of Medicare patients.

Coverage of renal disease constituted the first time a specific ongoing disease was singled out for coverage, and concern over the overall costs of health care prompted Nixon to use federal money to bolster the creation of Health Maintenance Organizations (HMOs) as models for cost efficiencies.[38] For many patients with chronic disease, HMOs would come to represent restrictions on treatment and providers rather than improved access to health coverage at best. If Nixon thought HMOs might help control health care costs, he was wrong. Health care spending and Medicare and Medicaid deficits have plagued virtually all presidents since Nixon's time, and reached a pivotal point in 2010, when President Barack Obama helped push through the Patient Protection and Affordable Care Act.

It is not surprising that the move toward collecting more data to advance our understanding of chronic disease, toward the development of informed consent and codified research ethics, and toward expanded health coverage all happened in the decades immediately following World War Two. While the consequences of these changes are numerous, one of the simplest and most wide-reaching was the creation of a social distance between doctor and patient, and then hospital and community. As David Rothman describes, "bedside ethics gave way to bioethics."[39] This increased focus on ethics and collective decision making protected patients in new ways, but the social distance also created a gap in trust between patient and physician. Such a gap left plenty of space for the disease activists and patient advocates who emerged during the various social justice campaigns that followed.

CHAPTER 3

Disability Rights, Civil Rights, and Chronic Illness

WHEN Aviva Brandt, a forty-three-year old former Associated Press reporter, suddenly became ill in July 2007, she expected to either feel better quickly or receive a diagnosis for an ongoing problem. What started out as pneumonia, chest pain, and a hospitalization rapidly turned into ongoing, debilitating pain and fatigue, frequent infections, and other immune and autoimmune complications. More than four years later, she has undergone numerous tests and consulted with specialists in rheumatology and neurology and still has not received a final diagnosis that accounts for her extreme fatigue, diffuse pain, and various neurological symptoms.

"Healthy people don't understand how a person can be sick for months and years and have doctors still not know what's wrong with her. Some people get a funny look in their eye, like they think it must all be in my head because otherwise wouldn't I have a diagnosis by now? Medical science is so advanced, with all this technology and such, so how come good doctors can't figure out what's wrong with me?" Brandt asks.

She desperately wants a specific diagnosis, a URL she can pull up and recognize herself in. Beyond the intellectual disappointment of not getting an answer, more pragmatic questions plague her: Would her current medication regimen differ if she knew what was wrong? What else could she be doing to improve her health and quality of life? Will her lack of a specific diagnosis hamper her ability to receive much-needed Social Security

Disability Insurance benefits? And of course, there is the niggling frustration of how to answer the inevitable question directed at her from friends, family, and just about everyone she comes into contact with:

So, what's wrong with you, anyway?

Brandt's concerns reveal just how powerful—and, at times, dangerous—labels and categories are when it comes to living with symptoms. Some patients also take issue with the "illness" moniker itself, preferring the more benign "condition."

Dr. Sarah Whitman, the psychiatrist who specializes in treating people with chronic pain, finds such semantic distinctions critical.

"In my work, I don't use the term chronic pain patient, but insist on patient with chronic pain. It's a small difference in phrasing, but one that reflects what you see first—the disease or the person," she says. It's a sentiment that stretches across diagnostic boundaries. The term PWD, person with diabetes, is a common one in the diabetes online community, rather than the term "diabetic," as in "He is a diabetic." A person *has* diabetes; a person is not diabetes.

When I posed the distinction between illness, disease, and condition to patients with diverse health problems on my blog and in interview questions, responses ran the gamut: Some patients preferred to use "illness" because it was less scientific-sounding and clinical than "disease." On the other hand, other patients saw value in using the word "disease" since it conferred a type of validity and justification for their chronic pain that other words could not. For example, people living with migraine disease confront the claims their constant pain is "just a headache," much the way patients with chronic fatigue syndrome are told they are "just tired." (The rest of us get headaches and feel tired, so is what makes these complaints different simply a question of fortitude?) When I'm speaking about my health, I tend to describe PCD as a rare genetic disease, one that is somewhat similar to cystic fibrosis. The use of the word "disease" hasn't been a conscious one, but in retrospect I do see how the word offers some built-in credibility I didn't have when I was incorrectly diagnosed with "atypical asthma." Since practically no one has ever heard of PCD—including health care professionals, who, even if they have heard the term in passing, don't know much about how it works or how it is managed—I find the aspect of defining one disease by comparing it to another more interesting. Cystic fibrosis isn't nearly as common as, say, heart disease, diabetes, asthma, or arthritis, but it is more common and much more recognized by the general public than PCD is, so I leverage that familiarity.

"I tend to use 'illness' more than 'condition' or 'disease,'" Brandt says. "To me, 'condition' refers to something I live with that doesn't have much impact on my daily life. I have many allergies and asthma, but because they're almost entirely under control, I consider them a condition I have. No big deal. Sure, there's places, animals, and foods I need to avoid, but I've been living with that my entire life and it's second nature to the point that it's essentially something I deal with subconsciously."

I feel the same way about my thyroid condition: I take a daily pill, I check my thyroid hormones regularly through blood work, and beyond that, I don't give it too much thought. My medication controls the symptoms, and as long as I adjust my dosage when needed, it has very little bearing on the activities of my daily life. Naturally, the diseases that do incapacitate me and have regular, direct influence on my quality of life, my productivity, and my relationships are the ones I focus on; there is nothing as primal and immediate as the act of drawing breath.

Aviva Brandt also emphasizes the quality-of-life aspect in her perspectives on illness and her semantic choices. "My mystery illness, on the other hand, affects every single part of my life. I can't forget it or ignore it. It affects my entire family, especially my young daughter, who went from being home with mommy all the time to full-time daycare at age two and a half when I suddenly got too sick to take care of her on my own at home," she says. "I like the word 'disease,' and will probably use it if and when I finally get a diagnosis. But to me, the word implies that you know what you have. It's a scientific word in some ways. And since I'm in limbo-land, it doesn't feel like I have the right to use it yet."

Patients don't want to be reduced to a laundry list of symptoms or a disease label, yet science matters, and the words we choose to describe and categorize illness have enormous reach. A label *can* bestow many things: a medical billing code for insurance purposes; a course of treatment or medication; entrée to a particular community of like patients; validation for physical symptoms. On the other hand, the lack of a label or classification radiates complexity outward, too, from personal doubts and skepticism to difficulty securing necessary benefits or work accommodations. Ambiguity is often the enemy of patients.

The relationship between illness and disability is equally complicated. Not everyone with a physical disability has a chronic illness, and not everyone with a chronic illness is considered disabled by his or her symptoms; but there is a lot of crossover. Writer Susan Wendell makes a useful distinction between the "healthy disabled" and the "unhealthy disabled." The healthy disabled are those whose physical symptoms and limitations are fairly stable and predictable. She writes, "They may be people who were born with disabilities . . . or were disabled by accidents or illnesses later in life, but they regard themselves as healthy, not sick, they do not expect to die any sooner than any other healthy person their age, and they do not need or seek much more medical attention than other healthy people."[1] Population in this group is in flux, since some conditions do progress and, as Wendell notes, some people with relatively stable disabilities have other health conditions; but in general they are "healthy."

When I think of Aviva Brandt's ongoing medical and testing odyssey and the experiences of patients with diseases as diverse as multiple sclerosis to arthritis and many others, it is clear Wendell is onto something. People with chronic illness may not reside permanently in the land of the "unhealthy disabled," but many of us spend enough time there that we know this much: we do not fully belong in the world of the healthy, either. While people living with disabilities may not spend as much time actively "sick" as people with some chronic illnesses do, marginalization is often all too familiar.

"The metaphor that I keep returning to is 'curb cuts'; if you're an able-bodied person navigating a city sidewalk, you probably don't notice curb cuts, but if you're in a wheelchair they make all the difference in the world," observes Duncan Cross (not his real name), a thirty-something patient with Crohn's disease, an autoimmune disease that affects the bowel and gastrointestinal tract. "Lots of places used to build sidewalk curbs with total disregard for that fact, because they had no awareness of the wheelchair user's experience. Finally, folks in wheelchairs were able to get the message through—those three inches of concrete might as well be Hadrian's Wall, from their perspective. And most places started building their sidewalks differently as a result," he says.

With chronic illness, the solutions, like the symptoms, are not that concrete. As Wendell writes, "Many of us with chronic illnesses are not obviously disabled; to be recognized as disabled, we have to remind people frequently of our needs and limitations. That in itself can be a source of alienation from other people with disabilities, because it requires repeatedly calling attention to our impairments."[2] She's right: if you're part of a community that has fought for decades to gain footing in personal and professional realms, as the disability rights community has, then the experience of deliberately naming problems and (necessarily) demanding recognition and accommodations for them could run contrary to those goals. The unpredictability of symptoms and their severity that sets chronic illness apart from certain physical disabilities can also make for "unreliable activists," individuals who might be able to run workshops or attend policy meetings one day and be bedridden the very next.[3]

"There's not a similar awareness of the challenges facing sick people, nor a sense that people with chronic illness should be able—that positive action should be taken to encourage them—to participate in society," Cross says. When he was an undergraduate, his college had a scholarship program for disabled students. Funds were limited to supplying education-specific resources. For example, a blind student could use the money for an optical scanner, or a deaf student could hire someone to transcribe lectures. Though these services are important and useful, the scholarship program didn't address the needs of patients who might be disabled by chronic illness in the same way.

When a person has a physical disability that requires the use of a wheelchair, cane, or other assistive device, he or she benefits from basic rules and hard-fought parameters that have been put in place as accommodations. This does not always happen as it should, but from college disability services to employment programs, we are more equipped to handle the needs of people with physical handicaps. However, the invisibility of many chronic illnesses muddles these basic ideas of what able-bodied looks like: a patient might not "look sick" if he or she has a congenital heart disease or advanced rheumatoid arthritis, but he or she could have needs very similar to those of the person with a more obvious physical problem.

With visible disability, noticeable symptoms are both cause for comment and discrimination as well as the "evidence" through which individuals can access resources and accommodations. With invisible illness, the very same lack of obvious symptoms that allows us discretion over when to disclose illness can lead to further isolation or alienation. As a college writing instructor, I've seen firsthand how challenging it can be to help students with chronic illnesses (as well as mental health issues) because the procedures simply aren't always in place to support them the way they are for physical disabilities. Also, if students don't opt to disclose their illnesses to me and don't otherwise look sick, I often don't know there is a problem until the student has missed several classes and is behind and overwhelmed— which jeopardizes his or her health situation further.

"There is a gray area between the disabled and the chronically ill. It is a different conceptual category," says Dr. Joe Wright, a resident in a Boston teaching hospital who has researched the early HIV/AIDS movement and patient advocacy extensively, and who regularly treats patients with chronic disease. "It's the nature of a changing condition versus a stable condition; chronic illness is not like disability in the sense that sometimes it's stable-disabling, sometimes relapsing-remitting, sometimes progressive . . . if you're talking to people with ALS [amylotrophic lateral sclerosis] who are progressively, relentlessly disabled, it has got to be different than living with stable spinal cord injury or relapsing-remitting multiple sclerosis," he says.

Furthering complicating the scenario, for some patients, the stigma of the word *disabled* itself prevents them from claiming ownership of the term, even if it might accurately describe their experiences. In her work helping professionals with chronic illness stay employed, Rosalind Joffe knows how important the language we choose to describe our symptoms is. While terms like "disability" or "illness" have varying meanings and associations for different people, Joffe says the most important thing to focus on is how that definition fits into a person's self-concept: is it a positive or negative force?

"Language evokes meaning," she says. She doesn't like to use the term "disability," in fact, preferring the term "debilitating," which often more accurately depicts the status and implications of her clients' chronic health conditions.

When clients use certain language or terms, she asks them what those words means to them, and how it feels when they are applied to themselves.

"Sometimes you have to really own these terms," she says, focusing on the intent behind using particular terms over others. Is her client trying to speak to a boss and communicate needs? Is it a discussion about necessary accommodations in the workplace? That is when these distinctions extend beyond self-concept into the pragmatic, when the internal associations of language have repercussions in the external world.

For Aviva Brandt, applying this language to her own life remains challenging.

"'Disability' has a negative connotation because it focuses on the things we cannot do that 'normal' or 'healthy' people can. And I'm hesitant to use it, despite the fact that my illness gives me many limitations, because my health problems seem so minor compared to the 'truly' disabled, like a quadriplegic," Brandt says. "There's a . . . sense of shame for me (and for many others, I think) about admitting a disability. I just applied for SSDI, and it was depressing and a little embarrassing to do so. I'm depressed about it because I prefer to live in denial that this is going to be a long-lasting or permanent condition. And I'm embarrassed because even though rationally I know SSDI is an insurance policy that I paid into since I got my first job at age fourteen, it feels like asking for a handout. Like it's trying to go on welfare."

Like many other patients, Brandt finds herself caught between the physical needs of her illnesses and the stereotypes and stigmas that surround notions of who is "normal" and who is not. Even when we know deep down that normal is always a relative term, many of us have days when we want nothing more than to just look or feel normal, to pass through the day in the presence of the healthy and go undetected—a visitor's pass into the kingdom of the well, if you will. We want people to understand, but in order to understand they need to be able to "see" illness in a meaningful way—and that type of vulnerability is extremely difficult.

In *Stigma: Notes on the Management of Spoiled Identity*, sociologist Erving Goffman explores the perception of self and social identity. He describes three different kinds of stigma: that which comes from physical deformities and abnormalities; that which comes from differences in individual character, passions, beliefs and lifestyle, or mental/intellectual differences; and that which comes from race, nation, and religion.[4] Stigma divides us into those who Goffman calls "normals" and those who are are not "normals," and often it is the perception of the stigmatized individual as an outsider that makes the difference.

Though attitudes about lifestyle, sexual orientation, and physical and mental disabilities have shifted greatly since Goffman penned his 1963 treatise, it is clear how these various types of stigma influence the modern-day experience of living with illness. True, we have come a long way since the carnivalesque sideshow oddities and outcasts depicted in Tod Browning's 1932 movie *Freaks* or in cautionary tales like *The Elephant Man*, but still stereotypes remain. People living with disabilities and obvious physical problems are acutely aware of how the able-bodied world encounters them, just as people who are morbidly obese know when people are staring at them, whispering, or making callous remarks. However, since many chronic illnesses are invisible, patients not only perceive differences between themselves and the healthy but must also navigate what it is like to fall short of perceived expectations because of their limitations. From the healthy-looking heart patient who gets grief for using a handicapped parking placard to the hard-working employee whose performance is lagging due to an acute flare of an autoimmune disease no one knows she has, invisibility affords many opportunities for alienation.

It is easy to brush off these permutations as merely quibbling over words, but from a quality-of-life standpoint, they matter.

Like Aviva Brandt, Duncan Cross has grappled many times with whether or not his disease makes him disabled—and what the implications of that classification are personally and culturally. "Plenty of chronically ill people refuse to think of themselves as 'disabled,'" he says, since doing so might be construed as giving up. "This is an unfortunate tendency: first because it reinforces the stigma against people who do view themselves as disabled, which is just an ugly thing to do in any case; but second, and more perniciously, it creates an expectation that we should conform to the norms for healthy persons."

"To tell somebody with active Crohn's or lupus or even diabetes that they're expected to behave like someone without that disease is absurd and cruel," Cross says. "And we do it simply because we're afraid of the stigma associated with the label 'disabled.' I was, at least for a time, guilty of this myself . . . I only really got over it in 2003, when I had a massive flare that fully incapacitated me for several months. At that point, I couldn't pretend I was anything other than disabled."

Yet for all the differences in visibility and even philosophy, disability and illness are inextricably intertwined. For example, once Cross was comfortable identifying himself as disabled, he could start seeing some of the benefits that membership to this community offered someone with chronic illness. Namely, he could tap into what he sees as a deep tradition of activism and identity.

"In a strange way, it helped me feel like a part of something," he says. Before he was willing to call himself disabled, he was stuck as a "normal" person on the outside and someone grappling with incapacitating physical problems on the inside. As what he calls a very marginalized normal person, he couldn't identify with normal people's lives, even though he was supposedly "normal" himself.

"Now I am a very mainstream marginalized person, and I feel a lot of solidarity with people who are also disabled (whether they self-identify as such or not). Whatever the stigma of being disabled, this is a better way to think of myself than aspiring to unobtainable normalcy," he says. Rather than serving as a sign of giving up, claiming disability gave him the freedom to carve out a life characterized by more realistic expectations, a situation in which he could find success.

"For me, personally, and maybe for others, I think the [disability rights] movement also provided a vocabulary that I can use to talk about the place of chronically ill people in society," he says.

The fact that people with chronic illness are having more conversations about workplace accommodations, or are more vocal and active in disease outreach and advocacy, or have a working vocabulary to discuss their needs and challenges is due in no small way to the obstacles people with disabilities cleared, and to the disability rights activism of the 1970s. At the same time the doctor-patient relationship underwent significant changes, traditional views on gender, equality, and diversity were also thrown asunder. Under common goals for respect, access to employment, and the ability to lead productive lives free from stigma, the disability rights movement unified itself in ways the chronic illness community has yet to do, even decades later. The legacy of those gains, though, has a very real presence in the daily lives of millions of us.

The Civil and Disability Rights Movements (1960s–1970s)

"People with chronic illness are now among the living, we can talk about it," says Cynthia Toussaint, whose complex regional pain syndrome (CRPS) and intense chronic pain classify her as both chronically ill and disabled.

"I notice it more because I am disabled . . . clearly we have come a long way; there are more accommodations than ever before," she says. With decades of health struggles to draw on, she feels that people with chronic illness, disabilities, and pain are more a part of mainstream society. As an actor, in addition to being the founder of For Grace, a nonprofit organization geared toward helping women in pain, she sees the breakthroughs, such as more plentiful roles for wheelchair-bound actors, as well as the ongoing challenges we still face when it comes to gender and pain.

"People with chronic illness were let out of the closet by the movement in the sixties and seventies . . . all this empowerment has certainly helped. We deserve dignity and respect and that movement has given us that," she says.

The disability rights movement Toussaint and Cross both speak to yielded small, incremental gains in the nineteenth and twentieth centuries and emerged in the 1970s as a cross-disability rights activism. This modern movement operated (and continues to operate) on the principles that "people with disabilities are human beings with inalienable rights and that these rights can only be secured through collective political action."[5] These principles parallel those of the civil rights movement and women's health revolution that surfaced during the 1960s. In fact, the Civil Rights Act of 1964, the critical piece of legislation that banned discrimination based on race in public accommodations and employment and in federally assisted programs, would serve as the model for the disability rights movement.

Social movement spillover, which Samantha King defines in *Pink Ribbons, Inc.* as "when new movements grow from the foundations of existing movements and borrow from their strengths and strategies,"[6] figures prominently in the dramatic shift in patient activism in the early 1980s, but it also speaks to the social turmoil and social progress of the 1960s and '70s. The idea that minorities should have access to the same opportunities and privileges as whites, and should be given the appropriate resources to help this happen, would translate when it came to evaluating the ability of people with disabilities and illness to lead productive lives in mainstream society.

For patients, an important step in the civil rights movement was Title VI of the Civil Rights Act of 1964, which prohibited discrimination on the basis of race, color, and nation of origin from federally funded programs. This paved the way for desegregation of hospitals, just as it did for schools and other welfare agencies receiving federal funding. In a commentary piece in the *Journal of the National Medical Association* in 1965, then assistant secretary of the U.S. Department of Health, Education, and Welfare James Quigley asserted that segregation is but *one* form of discrimination when it comes to the access and delivery of health services. He wrote, "Restricting the staff privileges of Negro physicians to treating Negro patients, avoiding the promotion of Negro nurses to positions in which they would supervise white nurses, assigning rooms on the basis of racial rather than medical considerations—these and other practices which are all too widespread in all parts of the country, constitute discrimination just as separate entrances and wards and the denial of services to Negroes constitute segregation."[7] He urged his colleagues to understand that compliance must be in both the spirit and the letter of the law, and painted a comprehensive picture of what true compliance would look like in a health care setting (emphasis is his): *all* patients assigned to rooms regardless of race, color, or national origin; *all* physicians given consideration for staff privileges; *all* facilities, such as operating rooms, waiting rooms, cafeterias, and lounges, available to all; and *all* training programs for professional development available to all staff.[8]

The civil rights and disability rights movements, though governed by different goals and objectives, share the common quest for dignity and respect that still characterizes many of the battles we see in health care today. More specifically, the move toward desegregating hospitals meant improved access to ongoing care for patients with chronic diseases. Remember that the gains in life-sustaining technology and ICUs in the 1950s and '60s resulted in more people starting to live longer with and "die longer" from degenerative diseases. For minority patients, the incidences of type 2 diabetes, high blood pressure, and infant mortality were alarming, and in response, civil rights activists set up neighborhood health clinics to start to address these health crises. These local clinics of the 1960s and '70s sprang up to address immediate needs, but they also spread an important message, one that is particularly prescient in light of current debates over health care reform: health is a *right*, not a privilege.

A major yet unrealized goal of the desegregation agenda was a push for universal health care.[9] The desegregation of hospitals did not happen instantly or seamlessly, but this move was a crucial turning point in the motion toward equal and appropriate access for all, something we still struggle with almost five decades later as the gap between rich and poor widens, and as minority populations still live with disproportionate rates of many chronic diseases.

Disability rights activists had secured several gains prior to the civil rights movements—schools and colleges for the blind and deaf, wheelchair patents and development, the founding in 1921 of the American Foundation for the Blind, the Social Security Act of 1935, which gave federal assistance to blind people and disabled children, and many more. They did so in response to a long-standing prejudice against disability. For example, the 1912 publication of Henry Herbert Goddard's book *The Kallikak Family: A Study of the Heredity of Feeble-Mindedness*, which tied disability to immorality and claimed both were genetic, further propelled the burgeoning eugenics movement. Such propaganda and hysteria gave way to massive abuses of human rights, from forced sterilization of people with mental disabilities to institutionalization.[10]

What the civil rights movement gave disability rights activists was a frame for their protests, one that resonated with American society at the time, a society very much in upheaval and attuned to sweeping changes in human rights. The frame borrowed from the civil rights movement "included the notion that places should be accessible to all groups; the notion that all citizens should be able to exercise their political power through the voting booth; the notion that discrimination in hiring, promotion, or firing was not acceptable; and the notion that separate facilities were inherently unequal."[11] Shouldn't people with disabilities expect the same rights?

By 1970, an estimated 10 percent of the population identified themselves as being disabled, but politically, they weren't organized in a visible, active group, and the social barriers they faced, despite specific disabilities, were still significant.[12] A precursor to the heyday of disability rights were the Social Security Amendments of 1956, which created the Social Security Disability Insurance (SSDI) program for disabled workers between the ages of fifty and sixty-four. In 1958, benefits were extended to the dependents of disabled workers. Another key goal was the pushback against rote institutionalization of developmentally disabled individuals. In 1963, President John F. Kennedy's address to Congress that called for a reduction in the number of mentally disabled people living in institutions and for improved measures to help them function in society was considered by many activists to be a de facto call for deinstitutionalization and for an increase in community services. When Cynthia Toussaint talks about marginalization and being "among the living," the roots of her observations stem from the push to bring people with severe disabilities back from (often inhumane) institutions into society's fold.

In what is considered the first true piece of federal disability rights legislation, the Architectural Barriers Act of 1968 was passed, stating that all federally constructed buildings must be accessible to people with physical disabilities.[13] By now, the parallels to the civil rights movement are obvious: regardless of race, national origin, color, or physical or mental disability, each individual has a rightful place as a productive member of society. Here we begin to see the "curb cuts" becoming a mandate, a literal physical entry point for people who previously had been forced to linger on the sidelines of society.

Proponents of disability rights began to realize the true power of the courts to bring about change. By 1971, court cases and legislative amendments focused on deinstitutionalization and on bringing those with impairments beyond blindness into workshop systems and improving employment options. More court battles in the early 1970s gave advocates fodder to push for the Education for All Handicapped Children Act of 1975 and solidified the courts as a meaningful avenue through which to enact changes in disability rights. Throughout the early 1970s, disability groups, independent-living centers, legal coalitions, and associations grew in strength and purpose, filing lawsuits, calling for change, and exposing appalling conditions of those living in institutions.

Each successful step added momentum and confidence to their platform, but frustration with the lag in implementing these key victories reached a crescendo. The benchmark legislation of the modern-day disability rights movement was the Rehabilitation Act of 1973 and its Section 504. Section 504 prohibited programs that receive federal funds from discriminating against otherwise qualified individuals who happened to be handicapped.[14] It also opened employment and educational opportunities on an unprecedented level for people with disabilities, ultimately paving the way for the seminal Americans with Disabilities Act of 1990. Disability rights activists saw the power of the legislation and through grassroots mobilizations made its passage a priority.

As groundbreaking as the Rehabilitation Act and Section 504 were, they were also time-consuming and expensive to enact, which gave institutions the time and excuses to delay adopting these policies. In 1977, mass demonstrations pushed for the implementation of the Rehabilitation Act and Section 504, which had been passed into law four years earlier. By this point in history, Americans were used to seeing protests: protests over voting rights and against segregation, against the Vietnam War, or for women's rights, for example. Never before, though, had groups of disabled citizens banded together in mass sit-ins and protests with such force. Sit-ins were coordinated in cities across the country, but the sit-in staged at the offices of the U.S. Department of Health, Education, and Welfare in San Francisco lasted weeks, with more than one hundred disabled protesters occupying the building until their demands were met.[15] The victory was, of course, an emotional triumph for the protesters, but it translated into so much more. What are considered "central disability rights concepts" (such as reasonable modification, reasonable accommodation, and undue burden) became the foundation for future federal laws involving disability and employment, and stem from the events of 1977.[16]

Barbara Kivowitz wasn't a patient with chronic pain when she lived through the disability rights protests in the 1970s, but she appreciated the changes they wrought from a professional perspective. Working in the corporate world in the 1980s and '90s, she witnessed an evolution in understanding of disability and in considering employees as workers, not as people with disabilities.

"There was just a much greater appreciation of looking at people's competencies . . . and a commitment to making accommodations where needed," she says. "The disability rights movement had a huge impact over the course of decades. There was unification, there was not differentiation between blindness, paralysis, [etc.]," she adds.

"My perspectives are [from working] in Boston and San Francisco so they are a bit biased, but what I see at least in those areas now is that people are much more conscious and much more cautious about issues of discrimination. People who have more complicated requirements may not be hired as quickly as someone who doesn't, but that is very much a behind-the-scenes factor," she says.

This last statement points to a reality Kivowitz now experiences in her own daily life: her chronic pain is an invisible condition with significant influence on her ability to work when it flares. As an independent consultant, she has the flexibility now to stop working when her health demands it, but she knows from her corporate experience that this flexibility is hard to come by for many.

The unification she saw through the lens of the workplace is actually the most striking aspect of the disability rights movement: the abandonment of impairment-specific agendas for more universal gains.

Previously, specific disability groups focused on equally specific goals and entitlements, rather than trying to change the terms through which society viewed all people with disabilities. The American Coalition of Citizens with Disabilities was founded in 1975 and became the "preeminent national, cross-disability rights organization of the 1970s," uniting disability groups who represented a broad spectrum of disabilities.[17]

"People with disabilities finally recognized the power in unity," Dr. Joe Wright says. When disability rights activists staged a massive sit-in in San Francisco, lobbied Congress persuasively, and brought their plight square in the faces of those who would be content to ignore them, they ushered in a new era of a more unified, more militant movement. For those living with chronic illness and looking for more societal support and accommodation, this angle of the disability rights movement is the most resonant.

"If there were people lying down in the streets in front of Congress it would be different," he says, reflecting on the comparison between the fight in 1977 for the implementation of Section 504 of the Rehabilitation Act of 1973 and the lack of such powerful demonstrations from the illness community during our most recent push for health care reform in 2010.

The disability rights movement's suspension of disease-specific goals in favor of broader needs is what differentiates it from chronic illness activism. "The political task of organizing around chronic illness, when there are people in so many situations and you have so many prognoses, is difficult," Dr. Wright adds. "I think there are even narrower categories you could conceivably organize around—pain, autoimmune disease, increasingly expensive biologicals. I have some sense that people with chronic illness need to organize but when I sit down and try to say, what is the agenda . . . it is not easy," he says. These divisions exist within disease communities too, not just among them: while some advocates push for a cure, others focus on making sure patients already living with a particular disease have the resources they need for quality-of-life purposes. In different circumstances and with disparate diagnoses, we will see this same division of focus and labor factor prominently in present-day experiences of illness.

Dr. Wright's assessment actually points to a much larger question for all of us affected by chronic illness: Is such mobilization even possible?

Disability Rights in a Modern Context

If the civil rights movement gave those fighting for disability rights a frame of dignity, respect, and equality, then the disability rights movement gave people with chronic illness a framework through which they could begin to address their particular needs and challenges. This frame applies to concrete matters of accommodations in the public sphere, but it applies to the more abstract, too. Suffering and isolation are a profound part of the human condition, and of all the commonalities illness and disability share, this is the most powerful. Susan Wendell writes, "Solidarity between people with chronic illnesses and people with other disabilities depends on acknowledging the existence of the suffering that justice cannot eliminate. It also depends on acknowledging that illness is not *only* suffering."[18] And she's right: living with chronic illnesses or disabilities means different ways of living, and, as she considers it, *different ways of being.*[19]

The Americans with Disabilities Act, signed into law in 1990, is the most comprehensive piece of disability rights legislation that exists to date. Its scope for the first time brought "full legal citizenship to Americans with disabilities." Under its auspices, local, state, and federal governments and their programs must be fully accessible, businesses with more than fifteen employees must make reasonable accommodations for disabled workers, and public places such as shops and restaurants must make reasonable modifications to provide access to people with disabilities.[20] When people with chronic illness sit down and talk to their employers to discuss ways to accommodate their particular symptoms and needs, it is the ADA that covers them and gives employers a set of legally defined parameters with which to avoid discrimination in the workplace. It is a piece of the legacy of the disability rights movement from decades earlier that has a tangible impact on people with chronic illness. However, just as legislation was but one part of the larger social adaptation toward people with disabilities back then, shifts in attitudes and associations are still needed to bridge the chronic-illness gap.

Some of the fundamental differences between chronic illness and disability remain obstacles. When the ADA was first written, disability was envisioned as a constant. A person's blindness, deafness, or mobility problems didn't fluctuate the way the symptoms of chronic illness do. As such, the ADA primarily accommodates obvious permanent impairments, rather than allowing for the fact that pain or fatigue may prevent a person from being able to perform certain tasks for periods of time, as is often the case with chronic illness. Rosalind Joffe takes a stance on this issue that she acknowledges some professional disease organizations and advocates view as an unpopular.

"I think you can't wave that ADA flag successfully. [It is] too hard to prove you have a case," Joffe says. Although employees should try to get what they think they deserve, issues of disclosure and accommodations are much more challenging when the problem isn't as black and white as permanent disability is. Still, what the disability rights movement and the ADA did do was at least open up the conversation, and given the complexities of chronic illness in the workplace, Joffe sees that as an important step.

The fact that more people are developing chronic illness (remember, nearly half the population lives with at least one chronic condition already) has made a dramatic difference in the lives of people with physical disabilities. The more these patients spread awareness, share their stories, and acknowledge the challenges that still remain, the more likely it is that some of these hurdles will dissipate.

"The stereotype of the pallid shut-in will give way to a broad panorama of styles and approaches," observes Duncan Cross. "We're going to have to learn to treat illness as yet another aspect of the wonderful and multifarious variation on the human theme, instead of as simply a problem needing a cure. Again, that's not to say that we shouldn't find cures and use them when we can—but we should not treat incurable people as unsolvable problems," he says.

Perhaps that sentiment above all others is the legacy of the disability rights movement for patients with chronic illness, regardless of diagnosis, labels, or employment. Even if we don't get cures, even if no miracle medication changes our situations enormously, even if we stay in Aviva Brandt's "limbo-land" permanently, we still deserve and should expect solutions to make our lives as productive as possible. The disability rights activism of the 1960s and '70s inevitably allowed patients with chronic illness to voice this. These activists' momentum also helped propel another movement with enormous influence on the lives of present-day patients: the women's health movement.

CHAPTER 4

The Women's Health Movement and Patient Empowerment

ALICIA Cornwell is a twenty-eight-year-old woman living with Crohn's disease, the same painful and often serious autoimmune disease of the colon and gastrointestinal tract that Duncan Cross has. When she first began her diagnostic journey, she was a middle-school student with stomach pains. She underwent a variety of tests, from endoscopies to barium-swallow X-rays, hopeful that each step would bring her closer to an answer and to some relief. While the tests and consultation initiated her into the world of patient-hood, they also signaled the start of an unfortunate but all too common cycle: dealing with the dismissal of her persistent symptoms. She was told she had reflux disease, but when her problems continued, so too did the tension. As the years went on, dismissal took on a more problematic bent, as physical symptoms were attributed to emotional problems.

"At that time, my parents and I were told that my symptoms were caused by stress. I heard this for years, right up until I was diagnosed with Crohn's [as an adult]. In fact, I had heard it so often, that until last year I was convinced I was making myself sick because I could not control my life, or, even worse, that I was making up symptoms for attention," she says.

This story line evokes outdated images of emotionally wrought, fragile women attended to with smelling salts and placed in darkened rooms that are ingrained in historical attitudes toward female patients—hysterical patients. The term "hysteria" originates from the Greek root *hystera* (which means womb), and it was once believed that hysteria was caused by the

womb wandering through the body. Victorian-era doctors attributed hysteria to an imbalance between sexual organs and the brain. "Problems that
we today regard as associated with hormonal fluctuations, such as PMS irritability and postpartum depression, were also prominent in the diagnosis
of hysteria," notes Paula Kamen.[1] The context for this Victorian-era belief
reaches back much farther in history; as we know, medieval perceptions of
women painted them as weak, inferior versions of men, and their monthly
cycles and hormonal fluctuations were catalogued as evidence that they
were mere leaky vessels, inferior to men in ways both physical and emotional. Unfortunately, this association between female hormones and character assignations is one that follows women well past medieval or even
premodern times.

The term "hysterical illness" often calls to my mind the narrator in
Charlotte Perkins Gilman's "The Yellow Wallpaper," published in 1892. In
the emblematic feminist short story, the female narrator's husband, a physician, barricades his wife in an attic bedroom, hoping that cutting her off
from the outside world and from any mental or physical stimulation will
cure her of postpartum depression, or "nervous illness," the catchall phrase
that is as disparaging as it is inaccurate.

"John is practical in the extreme. He has no patience with faith, an
intense horror of superstition, and he scoffs openly at any talk of things not
to be felt and seen and put down in figures," the narrator says of her husband. She further queries, "If a physician of high standing, and one's own
husband, assures friends and relatives that there is really nothing the
matter with one but temporary nervous depression—a slight hysterical
tendency—what is one to do?"[2]

In line with the plight of women throughout much of the nineteenth
and twentieth centuries, the narrator is physically and financially dependent on her husband. She knows that her forced seclusion only makes her
obsess over her feelings more, but she cannot escape. She is trapped by the
circumstances dictated by her social milieu and, accordingly, trapped by
the prevailing attitudes and (mis)understanding of mental illness and gender. For example, because early-twentieth-century physicians saw mental
illness as hysteria, little time or attention was given to actual treatments,

save the surgical removal of reproductive organs altogether.[3] Although "The Yellow Wallpaper" is a commentary on attitudes toward mental illness, its inherent points about the way female patients' needs are valued or undervalued resonate in conversations surrounding women and chronic illness.

For Alicia Cornwell, the doubt about her symptoms chipped away at her confidence, which, combined with her age—and the accompanying assumption that young people are not *supposed* to be sick—exacerbated the underlying problems even more. By the time she entered college, which is when she had what she now knows was her first true Crohn's flare, she was also experiencing a worsening of her reflux disease.

"Whenever I saw the university health center doctors about esophageal pain and the newer abdominal pain, they tended to focus on the reflux. I always felt timid around doctors (particularly men, which they often were), and my fears about my 'made-up' symptoms caused me a lot of anxiety when I needed to get checked out. Usually I minimized my pain because I didn't want to be perceived as whiny and weak. The fact that I minimized my pain made it even easier for doctors to routinely dismiss it," she says.

When she was referred to her third gastroenterologist for her first colonoscopy at age twenty-one, he told Cornwell that he noticed redness and inflammation but nothing that was cause for concern. He shifted blame for her symptoms to her lifestyle, not just her constitution. He told her that as a vegetarian she should eat better, and that she needed to keep her stress levels under better control, telling her that young women like her "often develop nervous stomachs and irritable bowel syndrome because of their stress."

Cornwell's frustration and indignation are familiar to me. So many times in college when I was admitted to the hospital, unable to breathe through my choking phlegm and narrow airways, my physicians queried if perhaps I wasn't just a little stressed out. I was a young college student who sounded even younger than I looked (I still sound that young), and maybe I just needed to learn to handle the pressures of work, school, and internships better. (No matter that I'd been balancing the demands of student life and illness since I entered kindergarten.) If they couldn't explain why I always caught so many infections, why all the steroids they pumped into me didn't control my lungs, then the causes couldn't be physical, right?

No matter how many times I explained that being sick and missing school and work was what caused me stress, rather than the stress causing my symptoms, I never felt they listened to that. Because of that resistance, they didn't consider alternatives besides histrionic asthma patient. Part of the reason bronchiectasis and primary ciliary dyskinesia are terms that carry so much meaning for me is because once I was diagnosed properly, I could start more appropriate and productive treatments. But getting those labels also meant I could shed the unwanted and interfering implications that because I was hard to diagnose (as most patients with rare diseases are), perhaps the problem was my emotional health. I don't think I saw my situation as directly related to gender at the time, and I certainly didn't make the connection to the broader struggle for women's health and patient equality. I was too busy living it, too busy trying to *survive* it, for any such introspection. It hits me now just how easy it was to pick up a file, look at a young woman with unexplained flares and exacerbations of symptoms, go through the cursory battery of tests, and then allude to stress when an obvious answer did not appear.

Cornwell and her current physician feel that had her original doctor not assumed it was her age and gender that were the problem, he would have done a more thorough examination and she could have been diagnosed and put on therapeutic medication years earlier.

"I didn't go to another doctor about my abdominal pain for several years, and I suffered a lot because of it," she says. Ultimately, it was a female nurse practitioner who listened to her symptoms and referred her to the physician who correctly diagnosed her and now helps her manage her condition.

For Janet Geddis, a young woman living with migraine disease, her age and all the assumptions that accompany it were also a hindrance in getting a diagnosis, but for different reasons.

"I've often felt that things were extra-tough on me when I was in high school and college suffering from migraine. I felt I was supposed to be happy, energetic, successful, and active all the time—and often, I was. I was very happy in high school and for most of college. The only dark spot on those times? My headache. Things may have been easier on me had I not kept the pain a secret. The majority of my closest friends had no idea I was suffering. Perhaps if I had been 'out' I would've received encouragement to go to a knowledgeable doctor and get a correct diagnosis," she says. "In ways, I didn't feel old enough or mature enough to have an illness that had to be taken seriously."

For many women living with chronic migraines, normal hormonal fluctuations can exacerbate or even trigger the debilitating headaches, which adds another layer of complexity to the relationship between gender and illness. Nowadays, exploring the link between hormonal changes and specific conditions is an important area of medical research, but remember this connection, because during the women's health movement of the 1960s and '70s, it would figure prominently.

"I have always been determined to not let [being a female] get in my way of getting what I deserve," says Geddis. "My mom was a member of the National Organization for Women (NOW); I was a self-proclaimed feminist starting freshman year of high school (but probably was one, at heart, long before that). That doesn't mean that others' preconceptions about females didn't affect me, of course—but I didn't suffer from timidity or shyness that women are often told, in not so subtle ways, to embrace in order to fit in. I'm not sure why it took so long to get an accurate diagnosis . . . I can't easily claim sexism there (as many patients do, and usually rightly so!) since [my doctor] was female. Granted, I realize females can be sexist, too. But you see what I'm saying, right? I probably didn't make my case clear; she probably did not ask the right questions. I have held on to a lot of anger toward her and other doctors I saw while I was a teenager, but I'm beginning to let that go."

Melissa McLaughlin considers lack of confidence to have been an instrumental part of her long, unproductive diagnostic journey. "I was a shy and quiet fifteen-year-old who brought her mother into every appointment (originally because the brain fog made concentrating and remembering difficult). They just didn't take me seriously in any way," she says. "Part of it has been my age; being young, shy, and unwilling and unsure of how to stick up for myself, I often found that I'd leave an appointment in tears, feeling bullied or belittled. For years, it didn't occur to me that I could argue with the doctor's results, even if they were contrary to what my body was telling me.

"I was a good girl—hardworking, a straight-A student, kind of a suck-up, even—and was determined to be a good patient, to do everything that they told me to do, because that was my only shot at getting better. I'd say it was about six years into things, about midway through college, that I finally decided that it was up to me, not up to them. If something was making me worse, I could stop doing it, even if the doctors told me I should keep doing it. If I could go back, I'd change that: that sense that they had all the control, not me," she says, honing in on one of the most important elements of female patient-hood: the balance of power in the doctor-patient relationship.

As a psychiatrist working with men and women in pain, Dr. Sarah Whitman reminds us that this imbalance of power and skepticism has far-reaching roots.

"Historically, when women have reported medical symptoms, these aren't taken as seriously as when men describe complaints. For example, research has shown that when men and women both report equivalent cardiac symptoms, men receive more thorough evaluations. And for equivalent cardiac disease, men receive more aggressive and definitive treatment. So a woman reporting pain may be more likely to be dismissed or [have] her distress downplayed," Dr. Whitman says. "There are some medical illnesses that are unique to women; for example, certain pelvic pain disorders. These are significantly under-researched, and it can even be difficult to find physicians with appropriate training and clinical experience to treat these diseases." The lack of training and clinical experience perpetuates the cycle: if women aren't diagnosed correctly because their physicians don't know what to look for, their symptoms worsen, which can have profound emotional effects on them, too. From there, it is not a huge leap to write their pain or symptoms off as hysterical or psychogenic.

In *The Camera My Mother Gave Me*, a candid, sparely written memoir by Susanna Kaysen—who also wrote the memoir *Girl, Interrupted*—

the author chronicles her journey toward an official diagnosis and treatment for her unrelenting vaginal pain. With each appointment and new remedy, from caustic creams and baths to alternative medicine and biofeedback, her frustration grows—toward the physicians who cannot help her; toward her partner, whose main concern is their lack of sex; toward her own body, which staunchly refuses to respond to her many attempts at relieving its pain. The more unsympathetic her partner becomes and the more theories are bounced around about the source of her pain, the more defensive and uncertain she becomes.

"Is this some way of turning against him?" she asks her alternative nurse. "Is this a hysterical illness?"[4] Not only is her physical condition in question, but her sexuality and her emotional state are, too.

"Just because we don't understand the cause doesn't mean it is not real . . . This is part of what's so bad about this disease. People feel responsible for it,"[5] the nurse tells Kaysen, who, of course, already knows this all too acutely.

So when it comes to pain, a steady companion of so many chronic conditions, why hasn't the image of the intractable female patient faded into the background of social consciousness or institutional memory?

"In a sense, women with chronic pain are in a 'perfect storm,'" says Dr. Whitman. She describes a potent combination of being in pain, being a woman, and especially having a "woman's illness."

Truly female diseases—those that, like Kaysen's, involve female reproductive organs—are even more mystifying and mishandled. The fact that these conditions are even less researched and understood adds to the combustion. Such statements certainly ring true for Barbara Kivowitz, who has undiagnosed pelvic pain. Kivowitz, as a fiftysomething consultant, brought the experience of living through the women's health movement to her doctor-patient relationship. Her journey was one of diagnostic exclusion, as likely diagnoses such as interstitial cystitis were ruled out, leaving her with unremitting, unnamed pain. However, like Cornwell and McLaughlin, she is a female living with pain, and that fact itself unites them more than their symptoms and diagnoses separate them.

As each one of the likely diagnoses was ruled out and Kivowitz still found no relief from the pain that left her homebound, feelings of power-lessness and helplessness increased. While she has had the somewhat anomalous experience of never having her symptoms dismissed outright—the result, she concludes, of a long-standing relationship with a wonder-ful primary care physician, excellent insurance, and above-average medical knowledge—she stills sees a worrisome dynamic when it comes to diagnosing and treating pain. The training doctors receive is "antithetical and almost hostile to this kind of treatment," she says, pointing out that most doctors are programmed to diagnose, heal, or say good-bye. The more resistant a set of symptoms is to diagnosis and the longer the process drags on—several years later, Kivowitz still lacks an official label for her severe pelvic pain—the more porous this system becomes.

When thinking about the challenging and often unsatisfactory expe-riences patients have had with physicians, Dr. Joe Wright sees part of it as the process of struggling with the power relationship that happens when we go to doctors. From the perspective of patients, they feel that "I had social power until I walked into this room." We see physicians when we are sick and vulnerable, and their assessment of what is wrong with us has the potential to validate or denigrate our experiences.

Activists have questioned the dynamics of what happens in that exam room. "There's this real tension about what we want from our doctors and [from] medicine," Dr. Wright says. "It is very hard for people just generally to make that individual experience political; it is what people with disabilities did, it is what feminists did, it is what people with AIDS did when each of those sets of people revised their relationships with their doctors." Putting individual experience into broader context enabled change to happen.

Their Bodies, Their Rights: Putting the Medical Establishment on Notice in the 1970s

The "perfect storm" Dr. Whitman mentions is an analogy that applies to the plight of the female patient for much of the twentieth century and pre-modern times. Women were navigating a hierarchical medical system dominated by males; women lacked knowledge and resources to advocate for their health, and they were saddled with the character assignations that women who are told "it's all in their heads" still see shades of today. Using the momentum of existing social movements, the women's health movement of the 1970s took specific aim at the traditional structure of modern medicine and the imbalance of power that put female patients at a disadvantage. The patients' rights movement discussed earlier was one catalyst for women's health activists, as informed consent in both research and treatment addressed the paternalism of doctors. The women's movement itself, an extension of the fight for civil rights and equality, was an important frame. As members of the women's movement, women's health activists "attempted to limit the extent to which the medical establishment controlled women's bodies and lives."[6] While the field of gynecology and obstetrics was a natural first target, activists sought to change the nature of the doctor-patient relationship across all specialties.

"The women's health movement said we are women and we count too, we have a choice when it comes to reproduction. We can have health, we can work, we have a choice," says Cynthia Toussaint, the longtime patient with chronic pain and a national advocate for women in pain. She was a teenage babysitter when she first read about Gloria Steinem and was hit with the realization that women were suppressed. In her own life, up to that point, she'd always believed women were cherished. That all changed at age twenty-one, when, after a ballet injury, she was struck with sudden, serious, unrelenting pain. More than a decade of dismissal and rejection followed. Despite being completely bedridden for long stretches at a time, Toussaint was told her symptoms were in her head, that she was crazy.

"What was so jolting for me was that I didn't get treatment for so long because I was a woman. Doctors flirted with me, they didn't pay attention [to my symptoms]. I needed help, my life was ending . . . my mom and I put it together early that it was because I was a woman," she says. She was ultimately diagnosed with CRPS and, much later, with fibromyalgia too, and she sees a lot of benefits from the work of 1970s women's health activists. "The women's health movement gave people with chronic illness a lot of credibility," she says.

The importance of the doctor-patient relationship in terms of women and chronic illnesses is significant. Looking first at obstetrics and gynecology, consider the millions of women who live with conditions like endometriosis and interstitial cystitis, or who live with infertility, which affects ten percent of (or 6.1 million) women.[7] According to the American Autoimmune Related Diseases Association, autoimmune diseases, which include conditions like lupus, rheumatoid arthritis, multiple sclerosis, and more than one hundred others, afflict fifty million Americans and strike women nearly 75 percent of the time.[8] A survey taken by the association found that 45 percent of patients with autoimmune disease were labeled as chronic complainers early in their diagnostic journeys, with the resulting delay in diagnosis often leading to organ damage from lack of appropriate treatment.[9] With just this small sampling of statistics in mind, the stakes involved in creating a sound, trusting relationship between female patient and provider are clear.

Another way to look at it is this: at the beginning of the twentieth century, the major causes of death for women were infectious diseases (tuberculosis, syphilis, pneumonia, and influenza). By the end of the twentieth century, those major causes had shifted to chronic illnesses (cardiovascular disease, cancer, stroke, and diabetes). This may seem like an enormous change, and in many respects it was, but the bookends share one fundamental characteristic: infectious diseases, cardiovascular disease, some diabetes, and cancers are often in part preventable.[10] We know much more about these chronic conditions today, as well as what we might do to help minimize our risk of developing them, yet so much that determines the diagnosis, prevention, and the course of illness lies beyond basic physiology.

Between the changes in medical and research ethics, the desegregation of hospitals, and the advent of Medicare and HMOs, health care was an increasingly large-stakes political issue in the 1960s and 1970s. A similar call to action to the one occurring for minorities, elderly, and the disabled during this era of social justice was taking place for women. As scholar Beatrix Hoffman observed, "Although each movement had its leaders, each relied on grassroots participation, or 'change from below': they were made up of ordinary people demanding reform, often on their own behalf."[11] The importance of this "change-from-below" aspect of reform in the United States cannot be overstated, as it not only propelled the civil and disability rights movements taking place but characterized much of the patient advocacy that would become so integral to the chronic illness experience. For example, in *Pink Ribbons, Inc.: Breast Cancer and the Politics of Philanthropy*, Samantha King connects the women's health movement's criticism of the patriarchal structure of medicine with helping build a foundation for the breast cancer activists who would soon follow.[12]

The women's health movement gave credibility to those with chronic illness, from the individual patient in an exam room who realized she had a valuable role in her health management and her relationship with her physician, to the various disease and patient advocacy groups that would emerge. Each can point at least partially to the work done by women's health advocates in the 1970s. While Congress and presidents haggled out agreements on Medicare and bioethicists and philosophers pondered the implications of life-prolonging technology and transplantation, it was patients, advocates, and those who felt they were treated like second-class citizens who empowered change. For women, this change started with the radical notion that they had a right to know about their own bodies, had a right to control their own health care, and belonged in medical schools where they could fully participate in the very health care decisions that have such significance in their lives. The grassroots women's health activism that emerged in the late 1960s and early 1970s was fostered by an equally diverse group of advocates, among them middle-class white women, middle- and working-class African-Americans, lesbians, and heterosexuals.[13]

Women's health activists shared the same type of vision for female patients, and the conversations surrounding what was possible, if not essential, for the doctor-patient relationship and women's health turned thoughts into action. The results were concrete and monumental. In 1966, the National Organization for Women (NOW) was formed. Part of the founding mission statement includes the aim to "bring women into full participation in the mainstream of American society now, exercising all privileges and responsibilities thereof in truly equal partnership with men."[14] The extension of those ideals of a truly equal partnership and full participation is a natural one, especially given the legal, scientific, and political shifts around women's reproductive health at the time.

The move away from medicalized pregnancies and births was one way women claimed control of their bodies. The practice of using midwives experienced resurgence in the 1970s, as women tried to create more natural settings for their childbirths and move them away from hospitals (which, as we know, more and more patients were spending longer amounts of time in by this point.)[15]

Women's advocates helped educate patients about the birth control pill, which was first available in 1960. When early versions were linked to increased risk of stroke, blood clots, and cardiovascular disease, advocates helped spread this information. In response to these concerns, the Food and Drug Administration (FDA) included with birth control prescriptions the first drug safety pamphlet written specifically for consumers that outlined both its risks and benefits.[16]

The landmark court case *Roe v. Wade*, which legalized abortion in 1973 by finding that preventing a woman's right to end her pregnancy violated her due process, was a pivotal piece of legislation in terms of reproductive rights, women's health, and women's ability to make decisions regarding their bodies. It was obviously a controversial ruling, one that also gave momentum to the right-to-life movement that proved so influential in the Karen Ann Quinlan case and to matters of life and death today.

One of the most influential and far-reaching conversations about what is possible for the doctor-patient relationship and empowerment and women's health took place in 1969, at an eight-woman conference at Emmanuel College in Boston. The paternalism of modern medicine was renounced in favor of finding practitioners willing to share their expertise, and the women, who called themselves "the doctors group," took on the task of researching as much as they could about women's anatomy and physiology, venereal diseases, pregnancy, menopause, and nutrition.[17] This ultimately developed into the first printing of the epochal *Women and Their Bodies* in 1970. Filled with information on pregnancy, menopause, sexually transmitted disease, female anatomy and physiology, and other topics, the retitled *Our Bodies, Ourselves* went on to sell millions of copies and embodies the grassroots ideal that women should have access to and understanding of what goes on in their bodies.[18] Here again the "ground-up" nature of the movement is apparent: women researching relevant health matters and sharing that information with other women. This was no dry, medical tome written by ob-gyns.

As Sheryl Ruzek writes, the book's success and reach "really lies in the powerful combination of presenting solid evidence framed in terms of self-determination, patients' rights and social justice through women's own voices. Women's experience, not professional opinion, made this ground-breaking volume so powerful. While its appeal has always been its useful-ness as a source of personal health information, it continues to confront the politics of women's health."[19] With education and knowledge, women could more easily ask questions, understand diagnoses and terms, and as-sert themselves when it came time to discuss treatments and outcomes.

The self-health groups and consumer advocacy groups that emerged during this time, which shared many ideals common with *Our Bodies, Ourselves*, helped transform patients into more active consumers of health care. The collective decision making we hold as an integral part of health care today is an offshoot of the brand of health communication that made *Our Bodies, Ourselves* so successful.[20] In targeting the predominantly male establishment of medicine—and this included both medical education and the recruitment of medical personnel—feminists urged women to accept responsibility for their role in what amounted to an unsatisfactory relation-ship. The traditional role of the patient underwent enormous changes. The docile, "good" patient who did not question or doubt her physician lost favor to the empowered patient who expected proper customer service and treat-ment. Women were encouraged to seek treatment elsewhere should their requests for information or other needs not be met.[21]

Feminism challenged social practices in the doctor's office and recast relationships between compliant patient and infallible physician as part of the larger process to keep women down. It wasn't just gender that women's health activists challenged; it was also the politics of professionalism. The broader issue of how men dominated women became inextricably linked to the medical sphere and how doctors, who were predominantly male, dominated their patients.[22] Feminists at the time reframed the history of medicine as a history of exclusion: women excluded or discouraged from medical education, midwives excluded from the delivery room, and women excluded from conversations about their very health.[23]

For Barbara Kivowitz, the women's health movement has enormous influence on her modern-day experiences as a patient and her relationships with physicians. "I construct them along lines in which I require that I am an equal partner and that nothing is done to me or considered without my fully understanding and participating. I don't do it with fists raised or voice raised. In fact, I insist on constructing a relationship . . . One of the things I learned from the women's movement is authentic relationships with everything, and I bring that into health care," she says.

"I make sure right away they know who I am, I am an individual, and expect and require partnership. I don't come in with a manifesto, just who I am; I trace that right back to the formation I had growing up with the women's movement. If the relationship is damaging, then the outcome is not going to be a healing one. I've taught some of my providers what it means to be in a collaborative, partnering relationship. Partnership is two ways—I understand what I need and also what they need," Kivowitz says, foreshadowing the type of participatory medicine we see emerging today. There are several obstacles to finding this type of collaboration. For one, she is doubtful that medical schools teach the concept of partnership. For another, she has resources available to her that not all patients do. If she doesn't connect well with a physician, there are hundreds more she can consider. Living in an affluent area with numerous hospitals and having high-quality health insurance certainly makes finding the right fit much easier.

There have been both global and personal changes as a result of the activism of the 1970s. According to the U.S. Department of Health and Human Services, only 7 percent of physicians were women in 1960.[24] Due in part to strict quotas that limited applicants to women's-only schools, a gender discrimination suit in 1970, sponsored by the Women's Equity Action League, helped open up access to medical schools for female applicants. By the year 2000, nearly half of medical students were female.[25]

Between 1970 and 2005, women's numerical representation among practicing physicians increased from 25,000 to 225,000.[26]

"That alone changes the nature of health care and the doctor-patient relationship and direction of health care research. There is a direct line from the women's movement to this outcome and that's huge," Kivowitz says. "Having more women in health care, and involved in leadership in health care, changes what is considered illness. Look at chronic fatigue syndrome and pain—pain is now considered the fifth vital sign (along with temperature, pulse, blood pressure, and respiratory rate) . . . I think the women did that."

There was pushback from the medical community when redefining medical ethics and collaborative decision making when it involved transplants and questions of the right to die, and some within the medical community were reluctant to construct these new roles, too—roles that gave more control to patients. Clinics that used nonprofessional caregivers, offered alternative treatments, and relied on a message of self-help and empowerment were seen as especially threatening to the medical establishment.[27] Still, those physicians who supported the feminist critique of the medical establishment, particularly those involved in obstetric and gynecologic care, realized that women's health problems weren't merely physical. They were social and political,[28] as they had been in centuries past, and as they continue to be today. The various health movements of this era, from the establishment of local clinics to the organization of self-health literature and workshops, to the Patient's Bill of Rights—which clearly applied to the women who were often left out of the conversation when it came to their treatments—were natural byproducts of both social and political processes. In light of the history of forced sterilizations in this country, especially among women living in poverty and women who were minorities, emphasis on informed consent and patients' rights was an important component of the women's health movement.

Another focus of the women's health movement with long-reaching implications for patients with chronic illness was improved access to health care and health insurance. From the desegregation of hospitals to the establishment of alternative health care facilities, in various movements activists "challenged basic assumptions of medical practice in the United States, charging that it was not concerned enough with preventive and primary care. The most radical of these groups embedded their analyses of the political economy of health care in a larger critique of imperialism, capitalism, racism, and then, as feminist analysis developed, sexism."[29]

The funding of Medicare and Medicaid and the network of community health clinics it allowed for drastically changed the ability of the poor to receive affordable care, but that was just one part of a larger process. The women's health movement's perspective is deeply ingrained in the push for universal care. After all, as labor leaders and other activists brought to bear, employer-sponsored health insurance did little to help women, who at the time were largely employed in situations with no benefits: part-time work, contract and service industries, and, of course, homemaking. Beatrix Hoffman discusses how the collective that wrote *Our Bodies, Ourselves* argued against the profit-driven medicine that was responsible for unnecessary hysterectomies as well as the deaths of women with preventable cervical and uterine cancers who could not afford care. They believed that health care was a human right and should be provided to everyone—and given that ethos, any type of health care that relied on an insurance system for delivery was unacceptable.[30] Shades of the same argument exist today, as do the conversations surrounding fair and equitable delivery of health care.

An Unexpected Link Between Women's Health Advocacy and Pain

"Though other stereotypes bug me now and again, it's the assumption that I am in some way weaker and less capable due to my illness that drives me nuts (even though it's sometimes true). People without chronic illness cannot know what it's like to live with it every day; even when pain or other symptoms aren't present, they linger like ghosts, ready to come out of the woodwork when we least expect it," says Janet Geddis, the patient with migraine disease. "Healthy people don't live with these specters."

She echoes the sentiment expressed by many patients: unless you live with and experience the looming threat of symptoms firsthand, you can't possibly understand the emotional and physical toll of chronic illness. The healthy can no more imagine what it is to be sick than I can imagine what it would be like to be healthy and free from illness-related activities. It is simply not part of the life I have ever known, so I can try to picture what that would feel like, and how that would shape the decisions I made, but it is just that—a picture of what I think it would be like, not what it actually is. However inevitable, this division does set up a sort of "us versus them" mentality. Perhaps these differences are inescapable, but I think what many patients are searching for is common ground, an entrée into the world of the healthy. The healthy might not understand living with the specter of symptoms that could re-emerge on a whim, but that is not something people *want* to envision, either. The irony is that nearly half of us live with chronic conditions, and the data suggests that number will only grow. The same specters that haunt patients today will affect many of "them," too.

In the 1970s, women's health advocates didn't want these specters, either. Many of the stories in this book, and in the larger story of chronic illness, deal with chronic pain. It is an undeniable fact of life for millions of patients with diffuse conditions, particularly women. As we saw in the stories of diagnosis and doctor-patient relationships in the opening of this chapter, pain is at the root of so many of the conversations we have around illness and of so many of the tests and procedures we undertake with the hopes of better treatment. The pressing question remains, if the main focus and success of the women's health movement was redefining the doctor-patient relationship, then why are there still so many instances where women in pain have such unsatisfactory encounters?

It's a messy question with a complicated web of answers, but here are two of the most significant. First, admitting that pain and fatigue could be related to hormones or other gender and sex differences undermined the fight for equality that so many women waged in the 1970s. Research into sex-based differences in pain is only now emerging to help explain why men and women experience and therefore understand pain and illness in such disparate ways.

"Ironically, the women's health movement . . . generally has been apathetic, if not resistant, to the issue of pain and fatigue. In their efforts to counter enemies portraying women as essentially 'hysterical,' feminist thinkers have gone too far to the opposite extreme in denying chronic pain's reality, portraying it as mainly a tool of propaganda against us, a social construct," observes Paula Kamen.[31] So reluctant were they to be lumped in with the weak, psychosomatic archetypes of female patients throughout history that they completely distanced themselves from any position that included biological influence on fatigue or pain. The very existence of chronic pain, resistant to diagnosis—and potentially tied to female hormones—was contrary to the image of the strong, emboldened woman who was anything but a victim—not to her physician, not to her disease, and certainly not to her femaleness. This resistance makes sense in historical context, but given the current state of women and pain, it points to the need for a substantial redirection in how we address pain and sex-based differences.

The women's health movement changed the way physicians saw their patients and empowered patients to be more active consumers. Criticism of the one-way, paternalistic doctor-patient relationship spawned new, necessary discussions about patient autonomy and role expectations. These discussions were similar to the conversations taking place around informed consent, medical research, and quality of life and the right to die. The 1970s were rife with other social movements, including workers' rights and antiwar activism, but these particular social and political movements had both direct and indirect implications on health care and, ultimately, on chronic disease. Moreover, they formed the foundation for two of the most significant disease movements of the twentieth century: the early AIDS movement in the 1980s and the breast cancer movement. These disease movements demonstrate that the tenuous relationship between science and stereotypes and respect and resistance continued to evolve.

CHAPTER 5

Culture, Consumerism, and Character
Chronic Illness and Patient Advocacy
in the 1980s and 1990s

WHILE I shuttled from one pediatric specialist to another in the 1980s, I was only tangentially aware of the burgeoning AIDS epidemic, or of the fledging activism first initiated by the gay community that strengthened in power and broadened in its mission. I watched a movie about the Ryan White story and celebrated World AIDS Day for the first time as a high school freshman in 1994, but these events were mainly white noise in the background of my daily life. The 1980s were also the years when the modern breast cancer movement emerged from the smoldering recent history of the feminist movement and the consequent changes in how we perceived women's health and the role of the female patient. I was too young and too busy being sick myself to be aware of them, but the disease epidemics and the advocacy groups that developed in response to them would alter the course of the modern-day patient-hood that so many of us live every day.

Around the same time these Reagan-era patient movements gained momentum, each with its own political and social agendas, the first waves of patients with what would later be called chronic fatigue syndrome (CFS), or chronic fatigue immune dysfunction syndrome (CFIDS), showed up in doctor's offices. The trajectory of the "yuppie flu," which often affected upper-middle-class-white women, set its own course. For patients living with the invisible condition, it would be a different path from the one AIDS activists forged, but one equally susceptible to the associations many are quick to draw between illness, individual responsibility, and moral character. It is an association a large and diverse group of patients struggle under today, particularly in a time when "diseases of affluence" often dominate the political and social conversations around chronic illnesses. The relationship between our lifestyle and decisions and their medical and social ramifications is as problematic today as it was when first-generation AIDS activists declared foremost that instead of being called patients or victims, they were "People With AIDS."[1] In recognition of the social stigma surrounding their diagnoses, one of their first recommendations was that all people "not scapegoat people with AIDS, blame us for the epidemic or generalize about our lifestyles."[2]

Let's take a step back and consider the state of chronic disease prior to the AIDS epidemic. By 1979, chronic illness was perceived to be the primary health concern facing Americans, and by the late 1990s, the proportion of deaths related to chronic illness had risen 250 percent from the beginning of the twentieth century.[3] In Toba Schwaber and Lawrence A. Kerson's *Understanding Chronic Illness*, published in 1985, the authors focus on nine conditions that were among the most prevalent at the time: diabetes, heart disease, stroke, cancer, arthritis, respiratory disease, epilepsy, dementia, and substance abuse. As incidence and awareness of chronic illness grew, it did so in the face of cultural ideals of strength, fitness, and independence that were increasingly hard for patients to meet. Kerson and Schwaber noted at the time that, "the ability to be spontaneous, to have boundless energy, to look perpetually eighteen years old, to jog, to dash here and there is the ideal."[4]

Likewise, in discussing the charity walk/jog-a-thons that emerged as popular fund-raising events for disease groups, Samantha King describes the mid-1980s as the era of the "fitness boom," when millions of once-sedentary middle- and upper-class Americans took interest in physical fitness. In the 1980s, she writes, "the fit body became at once a status symbol and an emblem of an individual's purchasing power, moral health, self-control, and discipline."[5] This idea is but a recycled version of something we've seen for centuries, from the fetid poor whose communicable diseases were considered their own fault, to the hysterical women whose psychosomatic symptoms were ascribed to weak character and the fragility of their gender. For people who contracted the mysterious condition that would become known as AIDS through lifestyle choices, and for those whose malaise and chronic fatigue could not be banished by simply powering through it, this emphasis on the body as a barometer of discipline and character was especially problematic. For people living with cancer, particularly women with breast cancer, the image of the strong, almost indomitable body influenced the concept of survivorship and empowerment, too: we didn't see cancer patients when they were gaunt and haggard from their chemotherapy. We usually saw them when they were upright, mobile, and participating in charity events.

This aesthetic ideal took on another dimension when enhancement technologies grew in popularity in the 1980s and 1990s: cosmetic interventions that had once involved removing moles or warts had morphed into more invasive plastic surgery and lifestyle medications. Combine this with the development of gene therapy to treat genetic illnesses in the late 1980s, and bioethicists who could see farther down the road saw a looming shadow: eugenics.[6] In the early twentieth century, it had been people with mental or physical disabilities who suffered most from the theories behind eugenics. Now, genetic disease, inherited traits, perhaps even gender could potentially become targets. The distinctions between something that needed to be treated versus something a person might wish to have treated, between what a treatment was versus what an enhancement meant, became increasingly important, whether in terms of ethical concerns or of insurance coverage and medical necessity. We see the influence of that distinction all around us today, if commercials for a medication that treats the "condition" of having short eyelashes are any indication.

All of this took place against a particular 1980s economic and social backdrop. Despite companies starting to outsource jobs overseas, more working-class Americans finding themselves without jobs and reliant on government assistance, and the nuclear family beginning to disintegrate, individuals were called to take responsibility for maintaining their own well-being and quality of life.[7] There has been a minor cult of self-improvement in America since Benjamin Franklin's self-help homilies, and during the twentieth century, this philosophy of self-improvement changed because it began to be measured against the outward success of others, too.[8] People want to stand out for professional and personal accomplishments, and most are loath to be noticed for what is perceived to be wrong with them. Self-improvement and the comparison of self to others offered little solace to patients with chronic illnesses, who could not wish away their debilitation by sheer force of will or exercise, who often used government assistance, and who needed help managing medical expenses. The Benjamin Franklin brand of self-improvement also implies a long-standing sense of self-reliance that people with chronic illness can't always ascribe to, no matter their desire.

"We subscribe to a mythos in this country of self-sufficiency. This is thoroughly a myth, in my view, but it leads to a general idea that people need to take care of themselves (even though the people arguing this point of view often benefit greatly from the labors and deprivations of others)," says Duncan Cross.

"As much as self-sufficiency may seem like a virtue, however, it's illusory and also antithetical to a more important virtue: solidarity," he says. When he hears people talking about self-sufficiency, what he hears is a refusal to empathize with patients who have debilitating chronic illness. Solidarity among patient activists of the 1980s was inspired by a response to stigmatization of people with chronic illness implied by the idealization of vigor during the fitness boom, the resentment of those who relied on assistance during times of economic need, and the pervasive attitude that physical illness is related to moral character.

"There is a sizeable minority in this country which believes either explicitly or subconsciously that people deserve what they get. If you're sick, it must be because you did something awful, or are an awful person . . . Obviously, relatively few people who have chronic illnesses did anything to create those diseases, and even those who did don't deserve the suffering that results," Cross says. In many ways, this is another version of the "us versus them" mentality Janet Geddis has pointed out and of the internal hierarchy of illness Emerson Miller first described. We start with the healthy versus the sick, but the divisions keep on going. Some people believe that if you do X behavior, you deserve Y consequences. For the same reasons that the biomedical model of illness popular at this time fell noticeably short, this myopic view on suffering and blame falls short, too.

With all this in mind, the 1980s and '90s were a crucial time in terms of patient advocacy and empowerment and, in some respects, were a continuum of the evolution of basic human rights and dignity from previous decades. AIDS, breast cancer, and CFS took on social manifestations as well as physical ones: we see HIV/AIDS patients stigmatized for having a disease that is visible for the wrong reasons (lifestyle choices); we see breast cancer patients who are embraced by society and consumerism as being more sympathetic victims of a known disease; and CFS patients (mainly middle- and upper-middle-class females) are viewed with skepticism and doubt because they are sick with an illness we cannot "see."

People, Not Patient(s): The Early HIV/AIDS Movement

The World Health Organization (WHO) has classified the early AIDS epidemic into three main categories: the silent period between 1970 and 1981, the initial discovery period between 1981 and 1985, and the mobilization period between 1985 and 1988.[9] Doctors first noticed an unusual type of pneumonia and other immune irregularities in a handful of gay men in California; by the time the first paper dealing with AIDS was published in *Morbidity and Mortality Weekly Report* in June 1981, 250,000 Americans had been infected with the virus.[10] Technically, AIDS wasn't named as such until 1982, and the first heterosexual cases were confirmed in 1983. On both coasts, these early years were already busy ones for the People With AIDS (PWA) self-empowerment movement. These patient activists realized quickly that they were fighting for their very survival and could not afford to be passive.

A fundamental characteristic of earlier health movements, like the women's health movement, was the idea that change was grassroots in nature, not a top-down movement propagated by those in power. The early HIV/AIDS movement is a striking example of this change-from-below: a patient population took on the same medical and political institutions that would prefer to overlook their plight. In 1985, Ryan White, a young boy who contracted AIDS through a blood transfusion to treat his hemophilia, was denied entry to school because of his disease status. When questioned if he would send his own children to school with a student who had AIDS, then president Ronald Reagan said during a press conference that "It is true that some medical sources had said that this cannot be communicated in any way other than the ones we already know and which would not involve a child being in the school. And yet medicine has not come forth unequivocally and said, 'This we know for a fact, that it is safe.' And until they do, I think we just have to do the best we can with this problem. I can understand both sides of it."[11] Reagan would ultimately reverse federal policy regarding AIDS by his term's end, mandating that all people with the virus, whether they were symptomatic or not, were protected against discrimination from any institution or organization that received federal funds. By 1988, the government was taking a more visible role in disseminating information about AIDS: every household in the country received an "Understanding AIDS" brochure, a shortened version of then surgeon general C. Everett Koop's report on AIDS.[12]

Unlike the majority of illnesses we've discussed so far, HIV/AIDS is ultimately fatal. Compounded by the extreme social stigma surrounding it, patients faced what Dr. Joe Wright calls a social death, too. "When you have a diagnosis that is fatal, people start thinking of you as if you are already dead or functionally dead, and people pity you and you don't have a voice in politics because you are already dead," he says. This social death was devastating to the AIDS patients of the early 1980s, who were already marginalized due to the stigmas surrounding homosexuality and the "gay plague." Psychologist Gregory Herek, who has researched and written about stigma, illness, and HIV/AIDS, notes that being infected with HIV is a defining characteristic that relegates the person to what he calls a socially recognized and negatively perceived category.[13] Compared to most chronic conditions, HIV/AIDS is particularly damning in terms of social stigma because it is a condition largely considered to be result of an individual's actions; it is incurable and ultimately fatal; and it is perceived to be a risk to others.[14] The fact that it first manifested itself within a much-aligned population made things much worse.

Out of that marginalization came the most concerted and successful grassroots advocacy movement in the history of modern disease. These early HIV/AIDS activists were in the fight for their lives, and their efforts led to some monumental changes in the way the health system responded to patients with HIV/AIDS: reductions in the price of medications to treat the disease, a significant increase in funded research, and more expedient drug trials.[15] They also took a comprehensive look at the needs of their fellow people with AIDS and fought against inequalities in health care, as well as against discrimination and injustices within the health insurance industry. From the daily realities of illness—medications and access to appropriate health care—to the development of less discriminatory federal policies, to more abstract gains, such as replacing fear among much of the public with compassion and understanding, the amount of change AIDS activists brought about in less than one decade is nothing short of incredible.

The neglect and lack of attention to the needs of people with AIDS, coupled with negative attention when it received any, lasted through the mid-1980s. Tellingly, it was only when the threat to heterosexuals became apparent that AIDS became more than the afterthought gay disease. Ulrike Boehmer, scholar and author of *The Personal and the Political: Women's Activism in Response to the Breast Cancer and AIDS Epidemics*, first heard about AIDS in 1982, when the prevailing sentiment was that traditional institutions were led by heterosexuals who did not care if gay patients lived or died. Boehmer, however, didn't see AIDS as first and foremost a health issue. "It was not the disease component of AIDS that held my attention; from the beginning, I perceived AIDS as a gay and lesbian rights issue, and that was why it affected me long before I ever knew someone who had been infected," she writes.[16]

Its decidedly political slant separates the disease from many others. However, in many ways, the message of early HIV/AIDS activists was a familiar one. It is no coincidence that the seminal Denver Principles of 1983, the first codified statement of rights for people living with AIDS, echoed the spirit of the disability movement, women's health movement, and the Patient's Bill of Rights first formalized about a decade earlier. Two leaders of the PWA movement, Michael Callan and Dan Turner, reflected on their work in the early 1980s and its roots, saying that "Part of the widespread acceptance of the notion of self-empowerment must be attributed to lessons learned from the feminist and civil rights struggles."[17] These early activists renounced victimhood and demanded to be called "People With AIDS," a people-centered semantic difference many patient groups still emphasize today. Their statements involved far more than simply the right for treatment or information regarding their diagnoses. They had to lobby against eviction from their homes, against job discrimination based on their medical status, against the isolationism and pariah-like status their disease conferred upon them.

The Denver Principles concluded with a request for basic human respect and the right to both live *and* die with dignity.[18] The Denver Principles served as a catalyst for the formation of the AIDS Coalition to Unleash Power (ACT UP) and for the patient empowerment movement for people with AIDS. Though ACT UP is still active today, AIDS activism shifted with the advent of protease inhibitors in the 1990s, the drug cocktail responsible for slowing down the progression of HIV into AIDS.

Dr. Wright comments that influential members of ACT UP were having dinner with Dr. Anthony Fauci of the National Institutes of Health and were not still mired in hashing out the etiology of the disease itself. This comingling was possible in part because they were involved in setting research policy. "They were not arguing about what caused AIDS and were not fighting on multiple fronts. They were ready to accept many of the terms on which the battle [was] being defined. The broader the agenda gets, the harder it is to find the enemy and fight to win," he says. This distinguishes early AIDS activism and patient empowerment from many of the same social movements whose existence paved the way for these early successes. Modern-day AIDS exceptionalism—the argument that it does not serve HIV/AIDS patients well to collaborate with other disease groups for common gains—partially stems from this. Hard-fought funding and research and well-organized political and social support institutions thrive because of their sustained, specific focus.

"People who don't come from that position object to singling AIDS out and [think it] should filter into the broader public health system. I think that argument is nonsense because without the urgency and hard work, none of this would have emerged," Dr. Wright says. "The political situation with AIDS is complicated because there is a lot of infrastructure and funding streams. From a sheer political calculation, it might be that people with HIV have the least to gain from making alliances with others: they are either going to bring others up to their level or get dragged down."

Given the circumstances in which AIDS advocacy emerged, AIDS exceptionalism makes a lot of sense. But how will it fare now that HIV/AIDS is seen more and more as a chronic disease?

While still mainly focused on the singular disease, AIDS advocates have developed a comprehensive scope in terms of issues they address that matter in terms of quality of life and survival: health care, medication, poverty, housing, gender inequality, racism, education.[19] Susan Tannehill, director of client services at the AIDS Action Committee in Boston, says that a lot of the services her organization offers are poverty-based, such as addressing housing problems and addiction treatment, and that having HIV compounds these problems for their clients. Culturally, white men are still often more empowered than other populations, and issues of gender inequality are still largely at play, too; Tannehill points out that clinical trials are still largely done with men and HIV medications are dosed based on men's body weight.

As the focus has shifted domestically, so too has the prioritization of health issues for some people living with HIV—yet another sign that from a physical standpoint, at the very least, the disease has evolved from a more immediate death sentence to a manageable chronic condition. For example, none of Dr. Wright's patients with HIV consider HIV to be his or her biggest medical problem. "Some of them have problems downstream from HIV, it has not made life easy for them, but when I think about them as their doctor, immune suppression is not the biggest problem . . . some have effects from meds, but if their biggest problem is hepatitis C or hypertension, they are not quite as urgent about being an AIDS activist or organizing life around that identity," he says. In fact, he conducted an informal poll of people with diabetes and HIV and they say diabetes, which requires constant vigilance and management, is harder to live with (unless the person is living with full-blown AIDS).

"If you were to step back, social stigma is very powerful but it is not the only form of suffering there is," Dr. Wright says. That idea that suffering crosses lines of diagnosis, gender, social status, and prognosis is not only the piece that connects case studies of HIV/AIDS, breast cancer, and CFS, but it is what connects patients across the disease spectrum. More than that, it is the equalizing variable between the healthy and the sick—if only we recognize it as such.

How Breast Cancer Advocacy Changed the Stakes for Chronic Illness

Breast cancer is a particularly interesting example of looking at disease through the biomedical model, where the emphasis is on cures and biological origin of disease, rather than on prevention of disease and societal contributions to illness. This preference extends to cancer research and funding, where the focus is on various surgical and chemical therapies and early detection. This is particularly evident when it comes to mammograms, which are often misconstrued as preventive. A mammogram does not prevent cancer; rather, it allows for earlier detection and intervention.[20] In 2012, researchers expect more than two hundred thousand new invasive breast cancer diagnoses alone. Clearly, earlier detection and curative therapies are important and urgent. However, true prevention is complex and multifactorial, and patients already living with cancer—and the side effects of its treatment—have diverse needs some advocates fear may get overlooked in the quest for cures and research dollars.[21]

Debate over methods of mastectomy and other treatments had existed since the late 1880s; by the 1920s, breast cancer surgery was the most common type performed in the world.[22] In 1974, legendary breast cancer patient and activist Rose Kushner pushed to separate her surgical biopsy from her treatment decision in order to have the time and opportunity to decide whether a mastectomy was appropriate. This bucked the long-established trend of putting women under anesthesia who wouldn't know if they had lost a breast or not until they woke up.[23] Before informed consent became codified policy for breast cancer patients, Kushner herself usurped consent when it came to her own body.

The 1970s also marked the occasion of the first national breast cancer organization, Y-ME. Founded by breast cancer survivors Ann Marcou and Mimi Kaplan, Y-ME, which was forced to file for bankruptcy in 2012, considered itself foremost a survivors' organization. The timing of Kushner's advocacy and fledgling breast cancer organizations was significant. The public announcements that First Lady Betty Ford and Happy Rockefeller, wife of then vice president Nelson Rockefeller, both had breast cancer pushed the disease into a more national spotlight, the same way movie star Rock Hudson's and basketball great Magic Johnson's HIV/AIDS disclosures would years later.[24]

Treatment progressed in 1985, when lumpectomies combined with radiation were found to be as effective as the much more invasive mastectomies.[25] The 1980s were also when the patient advocacy and cause-related marketing that are so familiar to us now gained popularity. The now world-renowned Susan G. Komen for the Cure and the National Alliance of Breast Cancer Organizations (NABCO) were founded in 1982 and 1986, respectively. Founded by Nancy G. Brinker and named in honor of her sister, Susan Komen, who died of breast cancer, Susan G. Komen for the Cure (once called Susan G. Komen Breast Cancer Foundation) has provided more than $2 billion for breast cancer research through its Race for the Cure and other fund-raising efforts and is the largest nonprofit resource dedicated to breast cancer in the world. Its name alone denotes its primary mission: supporting science to find a cure for breast cancer, as well as ensuring quality health care for all patients. It has not been without its critics, either. Most recently, in 2012, Susan G. Komen for the Cure made headlines for its controversial decision to pull funding for breast cancer screenings from Planned Parenthood, often the only resource for such screenings available to minority and low-income patients. Komen officials later retreated from and apologized for the politically influenced move, but the incident galvanized critics who have feared the foundation has strayed from its mission for some time.[26]

By the early 1990s, breast cancer activism developed into more grass-roots efforts: support groups provided information on treatments and social support, and patient advocacy groups emerged to help empower patients to make their own decisions.[27] The shared experiences among these groups evolved into what author and breast cancer activism expert Maureen Casamayou calls "collective entrepreneurism."[28] Many of these activist-patients were educated and politically skilled, having participated themselves in the civil rights and feminist movements of the 1960s. For these women, breast cancer was the occasion to move yet again from the personal to the political, something feminists and women's health advocates had been doing for years.[29] White women face the highest risk of breast cancer, though African-American women have a higher incidence at an earlier age. African-American women's risk of death is about one in nine, a statistic attributed to delays in diagnosis.[30] This question of health disparities is especially relevant in the context of the historical battles waged for impartial care for all patients. Women undergoing treatment for breast cancer cannot typically advocate until they are finished with rigorous treatments; at that stage, many are considered in remission.

Cancer activism is complicated by the fact that the disease takes so many forms. "This not only impacts the scientific logistics of developing effective cancer treatments," says Kairol Rosenthal, author of *Everything Changes*, advocate for young adults living with cancer, and a patient with thyroid cancer, "but results in splintered disease type factions all vying for a piece of the research funding pie . . . There is no formal body helping these groups to create a prioritized agenda based on variables of need. We lack the focus that the AIDS community had." For example, groups like Breast Cancer Action, who focus on potential environmental causes of the disease, have a worthy fight, but to take up the environmental angle means they are pitted against every major polluting industry. This does not mean it isn't a cause worth fighting, one that could yield a big difference for patients down the road, especially in terms of prevention, but it means less attention is put toward the needs of the patients already living with breast cancer. It is similar to the dilemma faced by those looking to isolate the environmental contributions to autoimmune disease, for example, which is a necessary and noble undertaking.

"[The early AIDS movement] was so successful because they understood well how to tackle public policy and government . . . Finding a cure for cancer is constrained by the limits of science, but insuring more citizens is only constrained by the human limits of politicians. The AIDS community was a tiny group adept at applying pressure to the government," Rosenthal says.

Breast cancer patients and advocates did not depend entirely on the political organization but also on the "informal alliance of large corporations" that helped grow public awareness of it. Pharmaceutical companies, medical equipment companies, cosmetic companies, major cancer charities, and foundations emerged on the scene and had the effect of launching breast cancer into the spotlight as one of the most well-known, visible diseases. In 1985, Zeneca (now AstraZeneca, manufacturer of the best-selling breast cancer drug tamoxifen), founded National Breast Cancer Awareness Month (NBCAM).[31] This was a precursor to what critics call the "pinkwashing" of America, as well as the growth of disease-specific awareness months and charity events, with their color-coded ribbons and symbols, throughout the year. Coming after the increased interest in fitness and activity of the 1980s, the time was ripe for the proliferation of sponsored charity events, particularly walk-a-thons and races. Samantha King writes that the "thon" is the product of a "specifically post-1980s, post-yuppie anti-materialism" that grew in the 1990s and underscored the need to feel fulfilled by doing something for other people.[32]

Now, breast cancer awareness month (October) is a cultural institution, with pink ribbons adorning consumer products in magazines, stores, and on television. The pink ribbon is "the most ubiquitous of these symbols, its presence on a T-shirt, a billboard, or a Hallmark card conferring an instantly recognizable set of meanings and values related to femininity, charity, white middle-class womanhood, and survivorship."[33]

The frustration some patients and advocates have with these types of events and cause-related marketing in general stems from the idea that gathering resources for research is important, but so are the emotional, physical, financial, and mental needs of those already living with illness. To augment Rosenthal's point, in its 2010 annual report, for example, Susan G. Komen reported that 2.2 million received breast cancer education courtesy of a Komen grant. Fifteen hundred breast cancer patients undergoing treatment were given financial assistance for pain and anti-nausea as well as other medical treatments and medical equipment via a different Komen grant.[34] "Many people defend the activity of raising awareness by saying, 'If this pink ribbon convinces one woman to do a self-breast exam then it is worth it,'" Rosenthal says. "Helping a single person to conduct a test that has not been proven to be effective is exactly how we will continue to lose the war on cancer." Despite smaller successes in treating breast cancer caught in the earliest stages, there is also much less attention paid to advanced metastatic cancer, which affects more than two hundred thousand people annually, with an average survival rate after stage IV diagnosis of only two to four years.[35]

While those within the breast cancer community have an essential perspective on cause-related marketing, so too do patients outside of it. From patients whose disease groups have embraced the ribbon/thon/awareness culture to those who live beyond the pale of it—some 25 million Americans like me who live with rare diseases and will never see our diseases become a touchstone—we are all impacted by the merger of consumer culture and survivorship culture.

Another potential consequence of cause-related marketing and activism is the expectations it puts on patients. What Samantha King calls "the tyranny of cheerfulness" is associated with many of these events. We know how comforting and necessary images of empowered survivors are. However, such emphasis doesn't leave room for people who don't see this diagnosis as a lucky gift, who aren't ready to point out silver linings—and, of course, for those who endured treatment and did not survive.[36]

In *Everything Changes*, Kairol Rosenthal writes, "the 'survivorship experience' has become a cultural phenomenon that is used to advance our disease on a national political level, to increase awareness, and to rally for needed psychosocial support services. Survivorship stories have also created a stereotype of cancer patients—even young adult cancer patients. We are seen as vocal, outspoken, sassy, sexy, insightful, spiritual, grateful, and empowered."[37] She told me she prefers the term "cancer patient" to "cancer survivor." As she described it, people who are not patients have this notion of finality—they latch on to what they know from popular culture. We want to put the most familiar vernacular on it, and people know the term "remission." People tend to think of a finish line that you cross as a cancer patient, she says, and all these pictures of people crossing finish lines in charity events perpetuate the stereotype of the valiant, effervescent cancer survivor. Within this paradigm, the long-term fear of recurrence doesn't get much attention, which she sees as a real problem. Plus, not everyone has access to the right treatments or gets diagnosed in time to have the survivorship experience our culture clings to tenaciously.

The issues apply to chronic illness in powerful ways. For one, there is obviously no finish line with chronic illness, literally or figuratively; we just live with symptoms that wax and wane and will continue to do so. Without that finish line that denotes survivorship, there is not the same level of cultural awareness or acceptance of our diseases, no backdrop of success with which outsiders can judge our journey. Our survival is more subtle and nuanced; it entails adaptation and negotiation, and is as fluid as our disease progression and symptoms are. It is this fluidity that Rosenthal sees missing in discussions about "surviving" cancer, and is part of the overall process of some cancers evolving into chronic diseases. The upside to this evolution, Rosenthal says wryly, "is that you didn't die." But living with cancer long-term, as she does with her thyroid tumors, is not a concept society has made room for as readily. It is a murky, gray space, when for so long we have thought about cancer in the static terms of living or dying.

This is not to say other chronic diseases have not benefited from breast cancer activism and, in particular, from cause-related marketing—or that there isn't true value and benefit in cause-related marketing's existence at all. In fact, it is now synonymous with much of the patient advocacy we have come to know. From arthritis to multiple sclerosis to lupus, there are numerous events that take place each year and hard-driving disease organizations that work to fund research and support services for patients. I have sponsored many walkers and runners, and I know that the community and energy they build are inspiring and helpful to patients and families and that alone makes them incredibly valuable. In many instances, funds raised can result in better understanding of treatments, new medications, or progress in the long journey toward a cure. I've done several benefit walks for my local children's hospital, where I spent much of my childhood, until my own symptoms made that more challenging in the humid summer months and I couldn't.

"I use the word 'slacktivism' to characterize the first decade of the twenty-first century when it comes to consumerism and illness. It is a given that cause-related marketing is in place to benefit sales and increase the profits of corporations while giving them a tax deduction," Rosenthal says. The "slacktivism" she criticizes, where we can click on links to donate or purchase products without any significant investment of human capital, has raised awareness for breast cancer and many other diseases, but ultimately, she views raising awareness as setting the bar too low.

"Two decades ago, when cancer was still somewhat of a whispered word, awareness was an important goal. But the cancer community has worked hard to achieve this goal and now needs to think about what are the next big steps. I think our next big goals involve starting to research causes and prevention, increasing access to life-saving drugs, and educating patients so they can take a more vocal role in helping to prioritize how funding is used so our research dollars can go farther," Rosenthal says.

Kathryn Ratcliff argues that breast cancer prevention—not just earlier detection, or improved therapeutic agents—would also entail a steadfast exploration of the environmental contributors to the disease, such as long-term exposure to hormones like estrogen and chemicals in plastics and pesticides. In a medical system that supports the biomedical model, where researchers and corporations and pharmaceutical companies all have their hand in the mix, making sure the needs and priorities of the patients come first is a challenging venture.

Invisibly, Impossibly Ill: Chronic Fatigue Syndrome

Paula Kamen writes about a particular subset of female patients whom she dubs the Tired Girls, sick with invisible illnesses (chronic fatigue, fibromyalgia, migraines) that in many cases have elicited doubt from health care providers. Melissa McLaughlin is one of the Tired Girls. She describes people who roll their eyes at her or come right out and tell her that CFS is a made up disease, a present-day hysteria, or that 'everybody gets tired.'

"Chronic fatigue syndrome is not the same as feeling tired because you were up all night studying for finals. Trust me," McLaughlin says. "It's hard to not have control over your everyday routines—to not be able to just go and do something without a ton of planning ahead of time. It's hard to live in . . . what I've always called the 'untils' . . . *until* something else goes wrong, *until* something improves, *until* there's a new drug that actually works for you, *until* there's an upswing in your symptoms . . . It's hard to see your peers doing things with their lives that you want to be doing with yours, and to know that you're just not physically capable of doing those things right now—or might never be. It's hard to be a grown woman and depend on your mother for a place to live, food to eat, the ability to take a shower or get to a doctor's appointment. It's hard not to figure out who you are now, now that you're pretty damn sure you aren't ever going to be 'cured,' but will always be a person with an illness," she says.

The phrase Tired Girls has stayed with me for years, because I know so many Tired Girls, because when some of my conditions flare, I *am* a Tired Girl who pays for the energy she expends, who must make calculated decisions about daily activities healthy people have the luxury to do without forethought or planning. The Tired Girl stands for so much that society disdains: weakness, exhaustion, dependence, unreliability, and the inability to get better. She is far removed from the cancer survivor triumphantly crossing the finish line in her local fund-raising event, surrounded by earnest supporters. The Tired Girls have few cheerleaders, and, often lacking correct diagnoses or effective treatments, wouldn't even know how to define what or where their finish line is.

Chronic fatigue sits squarely outside that biomedical model. Dorothy Wall writes, "There's no cultural representation for an enervating chronic illness like CFIDS. No valiant image, no stouthearted icon. You'd think, with the rising numbers of chronically ill, our cultural imagination would have expanded beyond the heartwarming and trite . . . What's disturbing is the elevation of accomplishment, its distillation into the moral equivalent of valor."[38] While the disease activism and agency of the 1980s into the '90s conjure up images of action—legislation passed, protests launched, funds raised, and miles walked—the concurrent advent of chronic fatigue syndrome tells a different story altogether. There are no pathology reports, surgical notes, or arsenal of chemical agents to treat it the way cancer is managed. There is no expectation of survivorship, partly since there is no cure, but partly since so many of us are quick to deny its existence in the first place.

It was the late 1970s and early '80s when a flu-like illness first began sending patients, many of them female, to doctors' offices around the country. Unlike the flu virus, it didn't go away. People complained of symptoms ranging from headaches and sore throats to brain fog and memory problems to muscle pain and, most significantly, profound fatigue that did not respond to rest. Unlike other infections, this illness didn't alter the patient's blood count perceptibly, it didn't kill them, and above all, it didn't go away. This transpired under what Wall calls the "dark undertow of AIDS."[39] With a lethal, infectious disease scaring the general populace and protest stories splashed across headlines, few had interest in a vague set of complaints about what many derisively called "yuppie flu," in a nod to the demographic most likely to suffer from it. Patients slogged on for months and years without significant improvement, and it wasn't until 1988 that the Centers for Disease Control and Prevention named the mystery illness chronic fatigue syndrome, a move that was not and is not without controversy.[40]

Some sociologists consider CFS to be a post-modern illness of our time. We favor constant activity, speed, and scheduled-ness that patients with CFS cannot adhere to, and often illness is blamed on these unwelcome features of modern life. CFS is not simply an illness, but a cultural phenomenon and metaphor of our times.[41] It evolved and spread in the community, making sense of distress by means of an acceptable narrative within the biomedical model. Once a set of symptoms has a label, critics suggest it heightens the risk patients will use the label to reinforce their sense of sickness.[42] Physicians often view the CFS diagnosis as a self-fulfilling prophecy, particularly when self-diagnosed patients seek their help.

On the other hand, many patients feel ascribing a label to these symptoms bestows relief, acceptance, and an end to the uncomfortable journey toward finding out what is wrong. Remember Aviva Brandt and her fervent hope to have a label, to be able to pull up a URL to describe her mystery illness to inquiring minds?

"There's a big part of me that fears getting a chronic fatigue syndrome or fibromyalgia label," says Brandt, "because those are diagnoses that are still controversial. Many lay people and even many in the medical community think they are essentially psychological problems; some even think the people who get those diagnoses are mostly drug seekers, looking for prescriptions for narcotics and other painkillers. So I want a label, but I want one that's accepted and acknowledged as a 'real disease.'"

As a patient with CFS as well as a researcher, Dorothy Wall experienced the skepticism as it unfolded. In *Encounters with the Invisible*, she discusses the "utterly dismissive" attitude of psychiatrists, medical historians, journalists, and cultural critics that prevailed for most of the 1980s and '90s. "From the disbelievers there are scathing polemics, a whole literature that dismisses patients as 'victims of sensationalist media propaganda and medical charlatanism' . . . The diagnosis of CFS is dismissed as breeding hopelessness . . . a cover for what is primarily psychological distress," she writes.[43]

What we now call chronic fatigue syndrome has appeared in various forms throughout history. It was often attributed to emotional rather than merely physical origins. One of CFS's best-known predecessors is neurasthenia, which was the term given to supposed "nervous exhaustion" in the nineteenth century. The term represented the belief that lack of strength in the nerves caused the overwhelming fatigue, and it was primarily a diagnosis of exclusion, when more obvious physical causes of exhaustion, like anemia, were ruled out.[44] Like today's chronic fatigue syndrome patients, many of these patients were female and upper-class, and many medical minds of the time attributed the malaise to the stress of increased educational and employment opportunities.

In the early 1980s, research into Epstein-Barr (EBV), the virus that causes mononucleosis, revealed that chronic fatigue can begin during a bout of acute infectious mononucleosis and, moreover, that some patients with chronic fatigue have unusual levels of antibodies to EBV antigens. However, researchers concluded that EBV does not cause CFS.[45] It wasn't until 1988 that researchers at the CDC called together clinicians and researchers to try and find some consensus on the issue. Since CFS does not have diagnostic tests, the definition was designed for research purposes and was made intentionally restrictive so that research studies could best detect associations between risk factors or laboratory abnormalities and CFS itself.[46] Patients had to have severe fatigue without another known physical cause for at least six months, and along with that needed to have at least four of the following symptoms: malaise following exercise, difficulty with memory or concentration, lack of refreshing sleep, muscle pain, joint pain in the absence of redness or swelling, swollen lymph nodes, and sore throat.[47]

The name itself has sparked ongoing controversy. One argument patients have is that giving a condition a name based on its symptoms and not its disease process can add to the misconception it is not a true disease. Moreover, attributing the bulk of the suffering many patients experience to fatigue does not offer a realistic picture of the quality-of-life issues and debilitation the condition can cause. The term "chronic fatigue" is readily met with the sentiment that "we *all* get tired sometimes." Patients try to explain that this fatigue is profound, overwhelming, and something entirely different from the tiredness that accompanies a long week at work, or the sleep deprivation that parenting a newborn entails. Part of the problem with the doubt many have about the condition and its psychological attributions is that depression and anxiety *can* cause many of the same symptoms. It is not unreasonable, then, to think that someone who is anxious and not sleeping well will feel poorly, or have trouble concentrating.

But what if the person is anxious because he or she has been sick for weeks or months and physicians can't seem to help? What if the person is depressed because he or she is at home sick, isolated from social events and falling behind in work? Who is to judge which comes first? This is why a concrete label and, more notably, a specific medical cause for the symptoms is so important to patients.

The controversy over the name exists within the patient community itself, too. One alternative name that is often used interchangeably is chronic fatigue and immune dysfunction syndrome (CFIDS). It alludes to the immunologic component many see involved. Some patients prefer the term often used in Europe, myalgic encephalomyelitis (ME). Since it points to a medically based explanation for illness (albeit one not supported by empirical evidence of brain or spinal cord inflammation, as the name suggests), many feel it substantiates the "realness" of their disease.

"Patients have led charges to change the name, to adopt the English term myalgic encephalopathy, but the CDC says that changing the name isn't a valuable use of their resources. Considering that a few years back they considered siphoning off funds set aside for the treatment of CFS to use for things like Alzheimer's, I'm not really sure that they are the best judge of how the public funds for this disease should get spent," Melissa McLaughlin says. In fact, after years of suspected misuse of federal funds ear-marked for CFS research, the CDC's program director for CFS, Dr. William Reeves, acknowledged the funding problem and asked for an official audit of the agency. The resulting Inspector General's report found that from 1995 through 1998, the CDC had inflated its CFS expenditures anywhere from 48 to 72 percent.[48] Though the funds have since been replaced, the years spent disregarding CFS in favor of other diseases put patients at a clear disadvantage and illustrates a built-in bias against the condition. In 2010, Dr. Reeves was reassigned to a different division, and one of his colleagues, Dr. Elizabeth Unger, replaced him. While advocates and researchers acknowledge a tone shift toward chronic fatigue syndrome with the departure of Reeves, it has been a gradual one, and more substantive progress needs to occur for them to feel confident in it.[49]

✿ ✿ ✿

It is not hard to see why early AIDS patients, who were fighting homophobia and intolerance in addition to a ravaging physical disease, faced stigma. Yet illness that is invisible through the lens of the medical science we've come to prize so highly is a cause for stigma, too. Though they emerged at practically the same time, the history of early AIDS is synonymous with political action and concrete results that the CFS community, despite the extensive work of disease advocacy groups and patients, cannot claim. Perhaps part of this is simply a question of demographics: AIDS patients were already marginalized in a way CFS patients were not, so the stakes were even greater. At the same time, it is clear why the iconic awareness and cause-related marketing breast cancer received in the 1980s and '90s does not apply to CFS. Remember, this was a time when self-reliance and physical fitness gained more prominence, when questions of character and moral integrity were mixed up with issues of economic well-being and philanthropy. If chronic illness in general is impervious to the concept of a finish line or a valiant victory, then one as subjective as chronic fatigue syndrome is that much more at odds with this projected ideal.

Patients with conditions like chronic fatigue syndrome occupy a frustrating space in the medical landscape, similar to that of patients with fibromyalgia, irritable bowel syndrome, migraine and chronic daily headache, and other concomitant conditions. The ability of medical science to reliably identify physiological, neurological, and biological causes of these conditions is critical to better acceptance and better treatment options. If we know what causes some of these invisible illnesses, perhaps someday they can be prevented. This is another reason why the emergence of a particular condition (CFS) at a particular time (the 1980s) has a far-reaching impact on the evolution of chronic illness in our country, the same way the growth of AIDS activism and breast cancer activism does.

CHAPTER 6

A Slight Hysterical Tendency
Revisiting "The Girl Who Cried Pain"

WHEN Cynthia Toussaint read the *New York Times*' January 14, 2008, front-page story ("Drug Approved. Is Disease Real?") about Lyrica, the drug approved by the FDA to treat fibromyalgia pain, her reaction to the skepticism put forth about the condition's existence was immediate and impassioned. In the first paragraph reporter Alex Berenson writes, "Fibromyalgia is a real disease. Or so says Pfizer in a new television advertising campaign for Lyrica, the first medicine approved to treat the pain condition, whose very existence is questioned by some doctors."[1]

"I was personally insulted and shocked. It hurt so many people, especially women," Toussaint says. She considers the condition's front-page treatment to be a reflection—an indictment, really—of how society views women: weak, vulnerable, and dependent.

"It took us back to the dark ages," she adds.

That Toussaint is quick to associate the Lyrica story with far-reaching implications for gender bias in chronic illness and chronic pain is not surprising. As the founder of For Grace, an organization dedicated to empowering women and ensuring equality in treatment for women in pain, she is professionally entrenched in the politics of pain and gender. She's also a patient whose pain was routinely dismissed for years, and is all too aware of the gender bias in treatment and diagnosis of pain.

Widespread pain conditions like fibromyalgia or chronic fatigue syndrome are especially social conditions, since their symptoms have a direct impact on a patient's ability to maintain various roles and identities. Ties to the outside world via employment, family obligations, activities and hobbies, and social engagements are whittled away, and physical and psychosocial isolation increases. Add to this process the fact that their symptoms and complaints are routinely viewed with skepticism from physicians, loved ones, or both, and the alienation of individual patients takes on more momentum. In *The Culture of Pain*, David B. Morris writes that pain "cannot be reduced to a mere transaction of the nervous system. The experience of pain is also shaped by such powerful cultural forces as gender, religion, and social class . . . Even when it just grinds on mercilessly, pain, like love, belongs among the basic human experiences that make us who we are."[2]

Given how many people experience chronic pain—some 116 million Americans—and how harmful and often ineffective painkillers can be, it is hardly surprising that pain is a hot-button research area.[3] Yet what makes pain a research field with so much pull is also what makes it almost impervious to quantitative data: pain is inherently subjective. Unlike blood tests that reveal certain abnormalities or X-rays or CT scans that reveal fissures, breaks, or masses, there are no universal, definitive tests for pain. Most often, the ubiquitous Comparative Pain Scale that asks patients to rate their pain from zero to ten (ten is the worst pain imaginable) is the standard benchmark. Pain is self-reported, and there is the fundamental problem: the person reporting it must be beyond skepticism, hesitation, or bias. While many would like to believe we've abandoned the days of hysterical illness and great strides have been made in the realm of sex-based research and understanding of psychosocial and biological differences in the perception and experience of pain, the female patient still confronts bias. If she is a patient of lower socioeconomic status, the difference is even more pronounced.

Research is beginning to show some promising information in terms of the perception and manifestation of pain between the sexes, data that could lead to more effective treatments and dispel the lingering stereotypes regarding both men and women who live with chronic pain. As it pertains to research, a person's sex as male or female refers to his or her

biological and chromosomal attributes, while a person's masculine or femi-
nine gender refers to the cultural roles and expectations attributed to that
person. We talk about sex when discussing research, since these biological
differences play an important role in the development and perception of
pain, but we more commonly discuss gender when referring to patients
living with pain. Sex-based clinical research that accounts for the differences between men and women is an indispensable part of more effective
treatments and improved outcomes. While much work remains, the changes
in research, policy, and advocacy that came about in the 1990s and early
2000s provided a foundation.

Sex Matters: Pain, Gender, and Medical Research

At its core, the Lyrica-fibromyalgia controversy has less to do with the
specific diagnosis and all to do with the nature of pain itself. Of all the
symptoms that manifest from chronic ailments, pain is the most frequent
unwelcome accompaniment. An estimated 25 percent of the population
lives in chronic pain, and it accounts for more than 20 percent of visits to
physicians. According to the Chronic Pain Research Alliance, inadequate
physician training and education in diagnosing and treating just six of
these pain disorders—fibromyalgia, chronic fatigue syndrome, endometriosis, interstitial cystitis, temporomandibular joint disorder (TMJ), and
vulvodynia, which affect 50 million women—adds as much as $80 billion
in both direct and indirect costs annually.[4] From multiple doctor visits to
lost wages and productivity due to flares, chronic pain is an expensive, exhausting endeavor.

Chronic pain, especially severe chronic pain, is so encompassing and
omnipresent it makes concentrating on anything else other than it nearly
impossible. Chronic pain can make it excruciating to engage in physical
activities, keep up with a regular work schedule, or even leave the house.
Over time, chronic pain erodes so many aspects of the patient's identity
that sometimes it seems all that is left is the minute-by-minute experience
of simply surviving the pain itself. It makes the threads of everyday life

blurry and out-of-reach, yet pain becomes the narrow, sharp lens through which everything else that matters is filtered. This is the reality behind the statistics, the jobs left behind, and the co-pays for painkillers that invite as many problems as the fleeting relief with which they tempt.

The women's health movement did a lot to change the doctor-patient relationship and the quality of life for women, especially those living with chronic illness, but it did not address gender and chronic pain. In fact, pointing out that women lived in pain that just might be associated with hormonal and other physiological differences between women and men was anathema to the push for recognition of women's equality. In what many consider the third wave of the women's health movement (with the Progressive Era in the early twentieth century and the women's health mobilization in the 1970s being the first two), the 1990s saw an increase in the number of female physicians and medical school students, and more female representation in Congress; ultimately, the federal government could no longer ignore the glaring disparities in sex-based clinical research.[5]

In 1990, the Society for Women's Health Research (SWHR) was founded. A collaboration by physicians, researchers, and women's health advocates, the organization's aim was to draw attention to the blatant lack of inclusion of women in medical research and trials supported by the National Institutes of Health and, specifically, the lack of research on the numerous diseases that either solely or disproportionately affected women.[6] To address inequity in medical research, the SWHR asked the Government Accounting Office (GAO) to look into the problem of sex-based research and examine if American women were truly at risk due to biases in clinical research. The GAO's report, released in June 1990, found that the National Institutes of Health's vague policy to encourage the inclusion of women in its trials was poorly communicated and not well understood in the research community, which clearly did not bode well for the millions of women depending on research to give them a better life.

By the early 1990s, chronic fatigue syndrome was already a contentious issue affecting many women, cause-related marketing for breast cancer was ramping up, and the iconic female survivor was growing more popular in public consciousness. The Americans with Disabilities Act (ADA), which prohibited discrimination in employment, transportation, and other public accommodations, was also passed in 1990. By the end of that decade, almost three-quarters of women of working age with a disability characterized as non-severe were in the workforce.[7] It was long past time for women's health and, in particular, women's pain as it related to chronic illness, to get recognition. A pivotal point came in 1993, with the passage of the NIH [National Institutes of Health] Revitalization Act, a law written with direct input from the Society for Women's Health Research that mandated women and minorities be included in all federally funded clinical research and that Phase 3 clinical trials to bring drugs to the market be analyzed by sex.[8]

The same hormonal and physiological differences between men and women that were problematic for women's health activists in the 1970s are especially important in terms of how medications and dosages work in male and female bodies. Once again at the request of the SWHR, the GAO stepped in to examine how the Food and Drug Administration (FDA), which has the discretion to approve drugs for sale and as arbiter of what passes muster for safety and quality, handled the inclusion of women in trials for drugs seeking approval for marketing to the public. The subsequent report found the FDA was not effective in managing the presentation and analysis of data in drug development that pertained to sex-based differences.[9] In response, both the FDA and the Centers for Disease Control and Prevention established Offices for Women's Health, another key step in the process toward better understanding, treating, and legitimizing women's pain.[10] The interest in sex-based biology and research continued to grow, and in 1996, the prestigious Institute of Medicine (IOM) received a proposal from the SWHR seeking validation of it and planning out the appropriate direction for research.[11] Another piece of the foundation was put into place when the ban on women of childbearing age from participating in early clinical trials, which had been put in place in 1977, was lifted. The ban was a leftover from the thalidomide tragedy of the 1960s and '70s, when babies of women who had taken the drug while pregnant were born severely deformed.[12] The lifting of this ban was a significant step, considering how many women manifest chronic and autoimmune conditions during their childbearing years.[13]

Sex-based research is a primary area of concern for patients, but it is not the only obstacle. The fact that physicians typically aren't trained appropriately enough in matters of women and pain is also problematic. This lack of education about women's health issues was given a boost in 1994, when the guidelines for incorporating women's health in medical school curricula were published, representing another piece of unfinished business.[14] This lack of awareness extends beyond simply matters of reproduction or chronic pain and influences the treatment of women across the disease spectrum. Dr. Sarah Whitman, the psychiatrist who specializes in working with men and women in pain, thinks some of the reason that women are treated differently from men is directly linked to this lack of knowledge.

"For example," she says, "women's symptoms of a heart attack are different than men's; if an M.D. doesn't know that, they'll miss a lot of heart attacks in women. Another example is that we used to think that women didn't get heart attacks until late into menopause—again, lack of knowledge—so a woman in her forties or fifties with either classic 'male' symptoms or classic 'female' symptoms didn't get evaluated [or] treated correctly. However, being seen as 'histrionic' causes women presenting with classic symptoms to be 'tut-tutted' and sent away with a pat on the head." Her example speaks to the complexity of the sex-gender relationship: biological differences are at play in the manifestations of heart attack symptoms in men and women, but gender roles and assumptions factor into the cultural interpretation of those physical symptoms.

"The intersection of pain and gender is fascinating. But first, I think it's important to understand how pain, and people with pain, are viewed in our society. The picture isn't positive. This is true even within the field of medicine, in addition to society at large. It's quite misunderstood," says Whitman.

"The Girl Who Cried Pain: A Bias Against Women in the Treatment of Pain," published in 2001 in the *Journal of Law, Medicine & Ethics*, is a seminal study, and not just for its extensive exploration of the literature surrounding gender and pain. Its title alone is provocative, setting its sights directly on the tenor of skepticism that pervades characterizations of women in pain. Part of the problem, as study authors Diane E. Hoffman and Anita J. Tarzian point out, is that the quest to isolate physiological differences between the sexes must also account for the other forces that are involved in the living experience of pain.

"The Girl Who Cried Pain" found that women's reports of pain are taken less seriously than men's, and they are less likely to receive aggressive treatment than are men. In fact, research shows that men who report pain are more likely to receive painkillers for their symptoms while women are given antidepressants and are more likely to have their pain dismissed as "emotional," "psychogenic," and "not real."[15] A female patient suffers constant, life-disrupting pain and is told it is in her head. She's given an antidepressant rather than a diagnosis or a painkiller, and her anxiety grows. As her quality of life deteriorates and her pain worsens, she becomes depressed. When she reports being depressed, her initial physical symptoms of pain are attributed to her depression. The farther along she goes without recognition or validation of her pain, the more distrustful of the medical establishment she becomes.

"One issue particular to pain medicine," says Whitman, "is the caricature of women as delicate, emotional, and prone to difficult-to-understand whims—in a word, hysterical. So it's easier to dismiss their pain complaints as 'it can't be that bad,' or, 'she's just overreacting.'"

Studies of gender roles and assimilation support and help to explain this continued phenomenon. Women still labor under the stereotype they are weak, and society still often employs the presupposition that men should be tougher and more capable of sticking out pain and illness, making them less likely to talk about it. For example, researchers found that from an early age, males are conditioned to regard weakness, vulnerability, or fear as worthy of shame and embarrassment, while women are acculturated to embrace more community-oriented expressions of pain and to reach out to social networks. Further, male study participants report experiencing an obligation to display stoicism in the face of pain.[16] Though she admits it is a generalization, Whitman points to the fact that men are more likely to withhold complaints of pain, but when they *do* complain, they are more likely to be taken seriously. Men frequently won't admit they're experiencing chest pain when they're having a heart attack, sometimes resulting in death because they did not get to an emergency room in time.

"Some of this is because they fear being 'wrong,' and fear someone will think them weak for complaining of something that's *not* a heart attack," Whitman says. Still, prevailing attitudes toward gender and pain work in their favor should they seek treatment. If men do go to the emergency department, they will receive quicker treatment since people will believe they have the level of chest pain they report: it's a heart attack until proven otherwise. She attributes some of this to the fact that even when the medical knowledge is there, it changes slowly and it usually falls on individual practitioners to keep up with and then incorporate new knowledge into practice. In addition, there's a lag between when useful findings are published or presented at conferences and when they're finally included as standard practice. Even more problematic is the fact that gender roles and expectations change even slower than medical practice.

Inevitably, this outdated model where men are stoic and don't complain and women are histrionic puts men at a disadvantage, too. Prior to the onset of his chronic fatigue syndrome in the winter of 2004, Eric X (not his real name) was more than simply a physically fit, otherwise healthy male. A member of the armed forces, he was in peak physical condition, and in his spare time, his activities included rock climbing, mountain climbing, cycling, and backpacking. In fact, just one month before the onset of the flu-like infection that kicked off his chronic fatigue, he had climbed a 14,000-foot mountain in Colorado. He certainly didn't fit the archetype of the malingering CFS sufferer that patients find so damning, and he was more surprised than anyone by his deteriorating health status.

"I would say the biggest bias I confront with the disease is my own. I was/am embarrassed to admit to anyone that I have . . . CFS. I was one of those guys who thought that CFS was primarily a disease of upper-middle-class white women! And to be honest, I can be very suspicious of anyone who says they have CFS. I'm a very practical and analytical person and if I can't see it, smell it, touch it, taste it or hear it, I have a hard time understanding it," he says. "My wife (a counselor) has been a big help in helping me come to terms mentally with my condition, but I still struggle. I only tell people who absolutely need to know, like my bosses and *some* friends. Initially, it helped a lot that people who knew me, knew how active I was, so they understood that something real had happened to me," he says.

His natural inclination to couch things in terms of what is "real" and measure that against his many physical accomplishments is telling. It is an internal tension that he describes, but it is not just that Eric expects strength and endurance from himself; as so many have observed, external pressure to live up to this is ingrained in our culture.

"I think my life experiences make it more difficult for me . . . I was high-energy. I traveled a lot and . . . had a lot of physically demanding pursuits. Those things significantly influenced my sense of self and my confidence. When I was no longer able to do those things, everything changed for me and I struggled," Eric says. Now a father, he says his family is "my reason for being on this earth, and I think that's what every man needs—a focus. So I kind of grew out of some of the things that made the fatigue hard to deal with, and they have been replaced with a family." Eric's emphasis on how losing those more physical aspects of his identity influenced his confidence and self-esteem speak to the truly social nature of chronic illness: as our ability to do the things that give us pride and identity diminishes, what is left to fill the void? For Eric, and many others patients I've spoken with, family and relationships did that.

As Eric's story illustrates, being active and productive are important elements of confidence and self-worth. For many, this translates into fulfilling employment. Cynthia Toussaint feels women's pain is also undervalued because historically, they have not been (and often still are not) the primary breadwinners. The reverse can also be problematic: men are primarily defined by their job and earning potential. As Dr. Sarah Whitman has discovered, when illness impacts their ability to meet these expectations, men's self-esteem can plummet. Since our society is one that places a high premium on hard work, status, and achievement, this is not unexpected. If you break down and report your pain symptoms but they do not improve and your quality of life deteriorates, you are a failure as a patient and as a productive member of society. This may also explain why men are found to wait longer than women to discuss their symptoms with their physicians. In that case, the same inaccurate stereotypes that paint women as malingering complainers put male patients in an equally hamstrung position: both are unable to adequately convey their needs, or their suffering.

There are greater complexities still. For example, the routine attribution of abdominal pain or symptoms to gynecological problems can delay or complicate the diagnostic process. A woman's age puts her at a further disadvantage in this respect. In a 2008 study in *Academic Emergency Medicine* designed to gauge gender disparities among emergency room patients complaining of abdominal pain, researchers found that even after adjustments for race, class, and triage assessment, women were less likely to receive pain medication than men, and those who did get medication waited a longer time than male patients for their medication.[17] For women under the age of fifty, these results were more pronounced, suggesting an inherent (though unconscious) bias against treating women for gynecologic pain and diseases, which primarily affect younger women. It's as if the existence of one type of pain, gynecological pain, precludes the existence of other (potentially emergent) sources of pain, such as abdominal pain.

Unless someone has lived with chronic pain or lived with someone who suffers from it, it can be difficult to imagine something can cause significant pain nearly around the clock. "That's improbable to many people. People assume patients are just complaining too much, not trying their best to get better," Whitman says. Lack of understanding from physicians is both an individual and institutional problem; even in the last years of the twentieth century, pain was not an established part of medical school curricula.

"People often underestimate how much pain I'm in because I don't spend a lot of time complaining about it," Melissa McLaughlin says. "Doctors seem to think I'm exaggerating my number scale of pain because if I *were* in that much pain, I wouldn't be functioning, they think. But here's the thing: I don't have a choice . . . my pain is my pain, and if there's going to be anything else in my life, I have to work through and past it, regardless of how high it is."

It's an untenable situation: patients are considered lazy or indulgent if they remain housebound, but should they manage some activity or productivity, then their pain can't be as severe and exhausting as they claim. Here again we see the contradiction so common in the social history of disease: the absence of outward physical manifestations of illness somehow negates the actual experience of having it. Rather than overreporting pain, as critics suggest chronic pain patients of all varieties do, McLaughlin and others cop to regularly *under*-reporting it, aligning them more closely with classic "male" stereotypes.

Those skeptical of fibromyalgia as a sound medical diagnosis argue these patients simply don't tolerate the normal aches and pains healthy people deal with and ignore and that they become fixated on every little symptom, cataloging their list of complaints. Dr. Frederick Wolfe, one of the physicians involved in the 1990 paper that first outlined guidelines for diagnosing fibromyalgia, which has not been linked to environmental or biological causes, counts himself among the skeptics. As stated in the article, he now feels fibromyalgia is "a physical response to stress, depression, and economic and social anxiety."[18]

Most patients would describe this relationship in reverse, meaning the physical pain of their conditions coupled with not being able to work and losing social relationships is what increases their stress and depression. This isn't too different from the same correction I had to make over and over in emergency rooms and ICU rooms when it came to my respiratory problems: not being able to breathe and being hospitalized and away from work caused me stress; stress did not cause my choking phlegm and constricted airways. Perhaps more than any other statement, Wolfe's makes fibromyalgia a preeminent case study in twenty-first-century social disease, the modern-day physiological equivalent of the "nervous" female patients of past centuries.

"I've definitely heard this response/'explanation' of fibro before, and have met its believers in person. They are not doctors that I go back to,"

Melissa McLaughlin says. "I've had enough of being blamed for my illnesses—So what if I was an overachiever? Guilty as charged—but I was not straining myself beyond any limits I'm aware of, not even compared to my own peers. I didn't have three jobs or need to get straight As. I did what I enjoyed, for the most part, and enjoyed what I did. I'm certainly not going to deny that my fibro responds negatively to stress, depression, and economic or social anxieties, but do I think they are the cause of it? I just don't. And I don't because I had none of those issues, not a single one, when I first got sick . . . I didn't have any more stress or pressure or anxieties than anybody else, and I certainly wasn't feeling overwhelmed by them," she says.

To McLaughlin, labeling her pain as the normal aches that healthy people learn to ignore, as skeptics have characterized fibromyalgia pain, is woefully inaccurate—and unfair. Yet it is something she deals with from friends and family, and especially from health care providers. In the years since she went from a normal, healthy teenager to an adult in chronic pain, she honestly can't count the number of times her pain has been dismissed, overlooked, or underestimated by a doctor: "Of course you're exhausted, you're working too hard" or "You can't still be in pain, that should've gotten better by now" or "I don't understand how your pain can be worse now than it was the last time I saw you," are common refrains. When it comes to the severity of her pain, the standard scale is a poor substitute.

"Telling them I'm an eight out of ten on the pain scale—on a fairly regular basis—doesn't seem to mean as much to them as it does to me," McLaughlin says. They're looking for static indices of disease, while she is looking for a way to lead a normal life, to leave the house, hold down a job, someday have a family of her own, to reclaim the social ties and roles her severe, unrelenting pain has taken away from her.

While some deny the existence of the disease and cast symptoms off as histrionic, others are less concerned with semantics and give priority to addressing lifestyle and medical interventions that improve symptoms. "There is no concrete evidence for a physical cause of fibromyalgia . . . and the patients I've treated have done well with increased physical activity, antidepressants, and improved sleep. Why is it important for people with chronic sleep deprivation (with body aches and irritability) to be given the label of 'fibromyalgia?' Is it for ease of coding and billing? For destigmatizing a mental health issue? Or for synthesizing symptoms into a syndrome with a name?" asks Dr. Val Jones, a rehabilitation specialist and founder and owner of Better Health, LLC, an online portal of health news and commentary.

Pain specialists like Dr. Whitman urge an integrated model of treatment that doesn't rely solely on medication and procedures but also focuses on behavioral changes, education, and advocacy. If we looked at chronic pain the same way we approach treating a disease like diabetes—whose regimen includes diet, exercise, and lifestyle changes in addition to medication—then perhaps we could begin to distance ourselves from the notion that if we could just "cure" chronic pain, we would be all set. In *The Pain Chronicles*, Melanie Thernstrom's fascinating exploration of pain throughout history, she writes, "The biological view of pain is in conflict not only with the way man through the ages has regarded pain, but with the way in which pain itself is *experienced*, not as an ordinary physical function, but as an extraordinary state of being . . . the biological model cannot explain the disconcerting flexibility of meaning in pain."[19] Pain is something that transcends a cure, a far more nuanced and complex entity than a collection of symptoms biology can address.

How much of this gap in diagnosis and treatment is also due to the assumptions physicians and patients bring to their relationship? Here is where the social cues and mores that manifest in the profoundly human interaction between doctor and patient exert their influence. Barbara Kivowitz is a well-educated middle-aged woman, a former therapist who is now a consultant. She is an informed patient and not afraid to speak her mind. Yet she noticed two significant trends in her encounters with physicians. First, when she described her pain, it was often in emotional terms—how miserable she was, how frustrated, how her severe pain impacted her life.

"I wouldn't hold back. I would assume that my experience of my pain and my feelings about it and intuitions about it were data. For a lot of doctors, that wasn't data," she says. In those moments, she detected impatience in her physicians' demeanor, a resistance to her display of emotions. Second, she noticed a dynamic when her partner, a male, joined her for appointments. He asked questions she would never think to ask, and approached things from an entirely different perspective.

"I do wonder if having the male in the room does automatically up the credibility curve a little bit," she says. She started talking about her symptoms differently, as if she were a scientist. First she had handwritten score charts of pain spikes and dips and would show the chart. She became deliberate and conscious about when she would release any emotion, and the release was controlled and put within the context of analytic data, establishing more credibility in her reporting.

Kivowitz's distinction between feelings and intuitions as data versus concrete numbers is particularly compelling in light of research that shows that men and women describe complex pain very differently. A 2008 study found that while women described their symptoms in vague, abstract terms, men used simple, concrete terms. Rather than illustrating how the pain influenced certain activities or emotions, men reported what hurt and where. As such, it was easier for doctors to hazard a diagnosis and then move on to the appropriate course of treatment for their male patients.[20] This research also fits in with earlier studies on gender roles and communication analyzed in "The Girl Who Cried Pain," which found that women were more likely to describe their pain within the context of their relationships and social networks.

Combined with previous data, these findings are actually promising. They provide a theoretical foundation for the fact that some of the reason women feel dismissed or undervalued when they seek treatment for pain isn't because they are inherently too emotional or too prone to complaining (as we know), but that they are "speaking another language." This is not to say that women are to blame for the lag in diagnosis and treatment. Rather, it points to some of the possible reasons why this pattern continues, and why physicians and patients alike should consider their modes of communication. Patients shouldn't be responsible for translating their subjective experiences of living with pain into scientists' terms anymore than physicians should be expected to extrapolate quantitative data points from vague impressions of pain. But if both sides have a better grasp of each other's needs and wants, then perhaps a middle ground is feasible. As David B. Morris writes in *The Culture of Pain*, "When we recognize that the experience of pain is not timeless but changing, the product of specific periods and particular cultures, we may also recognize we can *act* to change or influence our own futures."[21]

These findings also point to an important difference in the way both parties approach this pivotal interaction: physicians are interested in analyzing pain, whereas patients, many of whom have lived with pain for years, are less focused on the analysis of pain itself and more concerned with alternatives to their current pain management. When you consider the distinction between disease (that which can be quantified by tests and results) and illness (the subjective experience of living with a condition), this makes sense.

Toward an Answer: Pain in the Twenty-First Century

Like so many mythologies surrounding illness, the mythology of women in pain that has subsisted for so long exists in part because mystery still surrounds it. Pain and gender are irrevocably linked, so it is natural that addressing pain in an effective, comprehensive manner involves looking at the differences between the sexes.

"I'm an optimist by nature, but I believe there's evidence to support a hopeful outlook. The gains which will come soonest—which actually are occurring as we speak—are advances in the understanding and treatment of pain, regardless of gender," says Dr. Whitman. "One which will be crucial is a better *biological* understanding of pain—viewing it as a medical disease, rather than a psychological weakness. Because women are disproportionately affected by pain, this will benefit them the most.

"[Fibromyalgia] is one disorder where we've made recent progress. We have great studies using fMRI [functional MRI], which show that the brains of patients with FM react differently to painful stimuli, which points back again to biology. And Lyrica is a medication shown to be helpful in nerve pain, which supports newer thinking about FM being a nerve pain disorder," Whitman says. Continued research into the biological processes of diseases, including the role of hormonal fluctuations in the manifestation and perception of pain in women, are important on many levels, including treatment, quality of life, and patient validation and identity. The road is fraught with misfires and wrong turns, however. For example, in 2009, researchers thought they had isolated a virus (XMRV retrovirus) believed to be involved in chronic fatigue syndrome, but by 2011, a more comprehensive study disproved the association between the virus and the condition.[22] That same year, *Science* fully retracted an article that linked XMRV to chronic fatigue syndrome, due to contamination of blood samples and misrepresentation of data.[23]

A diverse and expanding body of research conducted in the 1990s found sex-based differences in risk of disease, progression of disease, responses to treatments for diseases, and overall outcomes of disease.[24] The focus intensified in 2001, when a groundbreaking report was published by the Institute of Medicine at the behest of the Society for Women's Health Research. The IOM study stated that studying sex differences could yield significant improvements in the health and lives of men and women, that research on sex differences should be conducted at every level in the body and at every stage of life, and that the research on sex differences should also include studying how men and women respond to medications.[25]

Why does sex matter so much, especially when it comes to disease and medication? For one thing, experts explain that sex is "both a phenotype and a genetically based bio-marker that may predict disease susceptibility, onset and severity or response to therapy."[26] We see this in terms of how many more women experience chronic pain and chronic pain conditions; but another example of this is cardiovascular disease, which affects both men and women but in men causes twice as many deaths.[27] In yet another area, while females are more prone to depressive and anxiety disorders, males are more prone to developing antisocial disorders and Tourette's syndrome.[28]

We must also consider the difference in average height and weight for males and females, which scientists call sexual dimorphism. Sexual dimorphism is related to differences in gene expression between men and women, and some of those genes whose expressions are different can also cause differences in the way we metabolize drugs and dosages. While men metabolize caffeine more quickly, for example, women are known to metabolize certain antibiotics and anxiety medications more rapidly. This means some drugs could work less effectively depending on the patient's sex, but in some cases, it also means women are more at risk than men for adverse—even lethal—side effects.[29] Hormonal changes in women may put them at more risk of side effects at certain points in their menstrual cycles than others.

This kind of information is extremely valuable to patients and physicians alike, especially the millions of women living in chronic pain, who may already experience changes in the severity of their symptoms and disease due to hormonal fluctuations. In a critical review of pain research published in the *Journal of Pain* in 2009, researchers found that "abundant evidence from recent epidemiologic studies clearly demonstrates that women are at substantially greater risk for many clinical pain conditions, and there is some suggestion that postoperative and procedural pain may be more severe among women than men . . . current human findings regarding sex differences in experimental pain indicate greater pain sensitivity among females compared with males for most pain modalities . . ."[30]

Those invested in pain and sex differences say that sex matters from "womb to tomb" and that includes how we treat pain—and how medications such as painkillers and anti-inflammatories work in our bodies.

"Just consider all the differences between men and women. At every level of the human body—the system, organ, tissue, cellular, and subcellular—there are a host of differences between sexes. Only recently have we started to understand how these differences impact the prevention, diagnosis, and treatment of disease. This underscores why physicians must have the freedom to prescribe the treatments best suited to the particular patient for whom they're caring,"[31] wrote Phyllis Greenberger, president and CEO of the Society for Women's Health Research, in a 2009 opinion piece in the *Boston Globe*. While the NIH Revitalization Act and similar guidelines developed by the FDA paved the way for the inclusion of women and minorities in clinical research, this has not yet translated into the type of analysis and information women need.

When I spoke with Greenberger, she said that the FDA knows there are differences between the sexes that matter and that while companies are required to include women in their studies, it just isn't being done on the scale it needs to be.

"There [are] lots of problems in terms of liability for certain conditions, and for the most part while the companies are required by regulations from the FDA to include women and minorities in clinical trials and they are supposed to be doing sex analysis, that part either doesn't get done or it doesn't make the label," she says. Some physicians know there are certain drugs within a class that may be more effective in men than in women, such as the SSRIs [selective serotonin reuptake inhibitors] that are used for depression. Greenberger points out that those medications don't have any labeling that gives instructions to women aside from a pregnancy label, which is the only thing that differentiates men from women on the label.

"The awareness is certainly there and the FDA and Office of Women's Health are pretty good about this and the inclusion is there in some cases, but the analysis and the transference to the labels just isn't there. There just aren't enough women in the studies for a statistically significant analysis of whether there are differences," she says.

Based on her experiences working with patients in pain of both genders, Dr. Whitman offers five specific steps she thinks can help society move forward when it comes to treating women in pain: improved education about pain in general; educating ourselves about our own medical conditions and treatment options; seeking a second or alternative opinion and questioning doctors; supporting organizations that seek to educate the public about pain or that support research in pain diseases; and advocating for increased research spending by the National Institutes of Health. She makes this last suggestion with good reason: while chronic pain is as prevalent as cancer, cardiovascular disease, and diabetes combined, the NIH spends 96 percent less on research on chronic pain than on these conditions.[32]

We've seen some progress. In 2011, the United States Senate called for an expanded and better-coordinated research effort for several pain conditions, including chronic fatigue syndrome, fibromyalgia, and endometriosis, and under the auspices of the Affordable Care Act, the NIH asked the Institute of Medicine to address the public health impact of chronic pain and come up with specific recommendations to improve how we research, treat, and understand pain. Approaching this report from a public health perspective inherently validates pain as a widespread, serious health issue.

Not coincidentally, many of the common-sense recommendations echo what the specialists who work with patients in chronic pain endorse. Among other things, the IOM report calls for the acceleration of data collection on pain incidence, prevalence, and treatments to better assess risk populations and trends over time. It highlights the need for better pain treatment that is tailored for the individual patient, treatment that relies on the self-management of pain by the patient, and treatment that includes collaboration between primary care physicians and pain specialists. It also recommends expanded education projects for patients, providers, and the general public that cover the "complex biological and psychosocial aspects to pain," including formalized undergraduate and graduate training programs.[33] The IOM acknowledged the strides made in understanding the "biological, cognitive, and psychological underpinnings of pain" and concluded that "the future promises advances in a number of fields—from genomic and cellular through behavioral mechanisms."[34] Still, the report points to gaps in research, particularly in terms of effective treatments, as well as in the funding, selection, and oversight of clinical trials. The report urges that these suggestions and problems be addressed and strategies be implemented by 2015. Time will tell how effective and influential this "blueprint for action" is in the treatment and comprehensive research of pain, but it is a start, and it opens up a more comprehensive view of pain as a multifactorial disease, not merely a symptom to treat.

As for whether news coverage of the fibromyalgia debate meant we reverted to the "dark ages" of pain and prejudice, the implications of past assumptions figures in the controversy. Female patients today are very conscious of the stereotype of the hysterical patient, so deeply ingrained is

it that it has become the characterization these patients fear most. Fibromyalgia and its other chronic pain counterparts are not psychosomatic expressions of social malaise but physical manifestations that have extreme
consequences for the social development of the patient. Recognizing their
social dimensions—the way we communicate, the expectations we hold for
ourselves, the irrepressible temptation to think youth equates health, for
example—allows for progress, physical and emotional.

The final element is the true biology of pain, but as we've seen, to say
the answer lies in sourcing the physical origin of the many conditions that
cause pain is just one facet of unshrouding the mystery. In *The Pain Chronicles*, Thernstrom discusses a newer paradigm of pain, a contemporary
model that "sees it as a complex interaction among parts of the brain . . . it
has also revealed the truth embedded in the nonscientific, premodern
model by showing the way in which pain is inherently meaningful because
it is not simply a matter of nerves firing, but an experience created by
meaning-making parts of the brain."[35]

Sontag's description of that "night-side of life," wherein the sick dwell
and which the healthy avoid, is especially fitting when it comes to those
suffering from chronic pain. Brain, body, heart, mind—severe and ongoing pain encompasses every aspect of a patient's being, fills in so many
crevices of his or her life, until it threatens to absorb them entirely. Since
the development, experience, and perception of pain are influenced by a
variety of factors, we should expect no less comprehensive an approach
toward researching and potentially treating it. Science holds the power to
at least partially demystify pain, but only if viewed within the context of
the societal norms that shape the individual patient's world.

CHAPTER 7

Into the Fray
Patients in the Digital Age

FOR Jennifer Crystal, a thirty-three-year-old woman living with Lyme disease and two of its co-infections, life changed dramatically with one tiny tick bite in the summer of 1997. It was the summer before her sophomore year at Middlebury College, and Crystal was working at a summer camp in Maine.

"I remember the day that everything changed, that summer at camp: I came into the dining hall after a long morning of lifeguarding, driving a ski boat, and chasing campers around in the sun. Suddenly the room started to spin. I got dizzy and shaky, and my hands were clammy. Everything seemed very far away, as if I were looking through a tunnel. The camp nurses immediately suspected dehydration, but when they heard how well I had in fact been hydrating all day, they realized I was having a low blood sugar reaction. That episode was the first of many, and soon I had a diagnosis of hypoglycemia. I'd never heard of it. It didn't make sense to me, or to any doctors, why I would suddenly develop hypoglycemia, but no one seemed overly concerned with finding the answer," she says.

It would be years before Crystal and her doctors would trace her symptoms back to that summer and to a tick bite, but as it turns out, that is not at all unusual when it comes to Lyme disease. The controversy surrounding the diagnosis of chronic Lyme disease and the schism it has caused between patients who say they have it and factions of the medical establishment who disagree with the diagnosis, symptoms, and treatment for it represents what is now a well-established pattern when it comes to chronic illness. In an article published in 1991, when Lyme disease was on the rise in terms of notoriety and diagnosis, physician and medical historian Robert Aronowitz wrote that "A market for somatic labels exists in the large pool of 'stressed-out' or somaticizing patients who seek to disguise an emotional complaint or to 'upgrade' their diagnosis from a nebulous one to a legitimate disease."[1] Aronowitz went on to write, "When one is not sure whether a patient has 'disease,' then both doctor and patient have room to speculate about the way in which life stress or other emotional problems may be expressed in bodily symptoms."[2] In some ways, this same formula can be applied to a host of readily identifiable chronic conditions in a familiar, rinse-lather-and-repeat pattern: patients report symptoms that are hard to explain, and a space opens up for questions and skepticism. The tempting answer is to let science clear up the confusion, since, unlike many of its contemporary illnesses, there is quantifiable evidence of Lyme disease.

Except when there isn't.

As an infectious disease, Lyme is more common than HIV/AIDS, and, in its own right, is as politically mired. It is the most common vector-borne illness in the country, meaning it is transmitted through a bite, and between 1992 and 2006, reported cases of Lyme disease more than doubled, topping at almost 250,000.[3] According to some estimates, up to 20,000 new cases are reported annually,[4] though some patients and physicians feel the numbers are actually much higher, since Lyme is often mistaken for diseases like chronic fatigue, fibromyalgia, rheumatoid arthritis, multiple sclerosis, and so on. Its politics, its patient advocacy community (which adapted quickly to the social media milieu), and its challenge to evidence-based medicine all make chronic Lyme disease a revealing portrait in present-day illness. Along with hotly debated topics like the association between autism and vaccines, these medical dramas have played out online in real time for much of the past decade, comments and postings often complementing or replacing altogether the protests of decades past. We saw in the last chapter how much science has the potential to bring understanding of the causes and treatments for chronic pain disorders. In the case of chronic Lyme and other chronic conditions, it isn't so much that the research is just emerging. Instead, often the research exists, but it is the strength of the science itself that is at issue—and technology helps fuel criticism and analysis, for better or worse.

In the twenty-first century, mobilization and protest often take place virtually, in that technology unites people with like ideas and like causes. The rapid, dramatic shift to a digital world has influenced how and where we work, how we spend our leisure time, and how we transform thought into action. Consider the Arab Spring movement in 2011: one man's self-immolation in December 2010 in response to oppression in Tunisia brought about protests that quickly spread through neighboring countries such as Egypt, Syria, and Libya. Technology like Facebook, Twitter, and Black-Berry Messenger helped protesters organize, helped the movements spread their message, and helped the outside world gauge what was going on. Stateside, the Occupy Wall Street and other Occupy spin-off protest movements in 2011 relied heavily on social media platforms to mobilize, voice their agendas, and garner support.

While digital advocacy has not turned virtual collaboration into in-person protest in the dramatic ways the Arab Spring examples show, it has still had an enormous influence on changing how we find, use, and spread information. For example, 80 percent of Internet users—and about three-quarters of U.S. adults use the Internet—have searched online for information on any of fifteen health topics, such as a specific disease or a treatment; and 34 percent of Internet users have utilized blogs, websites, and online news groups to read commentary about other people's health experiences.[5] As current-day controversies over diseases such as chronic Lyme illustrate, we've come a long way from the mid-twentieth-century hubris over medical science's capabilities. Instead of believing medicine and science can and will conquer most of what ails us, we're questioning it—and in turn, patients and advocates face increasing scrutiny, too. Now, virtual collaboration and information-sharing offer patients and patient-advocacy groups many benefits, but the flip side of this mobilization comes with a condition: the message must be accurate, and the information reliable.

Us Versus Them: Science as the Arbiter

For those living with chronic Lyme disease, the growth of the virtual world happened at a particularly fortuitous time. The short version of Lyme disease's incredibly complex story—truly, it is the stuff of long, extensively researched books in its own right—is that it often pits evidence-based medicine and quantifiable data against clinical observations and patient histories.

At least that is one external perspective. For those living within the quagmire that is chronic Lyme disease, it is a story of suffering and dismissal versus conflict of interest and corporate gain. Many physicians and the Infectious Diseases Society of America (IDSA) believe Lyme is primarily a short-term infectious disease that is treatable with a dose of antibiotics, and that long-term IV antibiotic treatment poses unnecessary risks and is not warranted. In fact, their position maintains that in more than twenty years of research, no convincing evidence exists to support the existence of chronic Lyme, and there is a lack of peer-reviewed literature supporting the opinion that the benefits of long-term antibiotics outweigh the risks.[6]

In 2007, the *New England Journal of Medicine* (*NEJM*) published a critical appraisal of chronic Lyme disease in which the authors wrote that "Chronic Lyme disease is the latest in a series of syndromes that have been postulated in an attempt to attribute medically unexplained symptoms to particular infections . . . the assumption that chronic, subjective symptoms are caused by persistent infection with *B. burgdorferi* [the Lyme spirochete] is not supported by carefully controlled laboratory studies or by controlled treatment trials."[7] The researchers and professional and public health organizations who do not hold with the chronic Lyme diagnosis do acknowledge what is called post-Lyme syndrome, which refers to longer-term damage to tissue and residual inflammation but does not indicate an actual ongoing infection.[8]

Dr. Allen Steere, one of the *NEJM* review's coauthors, is a lightning rod in the Lyme saga. He first identified the disease and traced its origin to deer ticks in the 1970s. A feature article in the *New York Times Magazine* of June 17, 2001, called "Stalking Dr. Steere over Lyme Disease" found that between 1982 and 1992, nearly 50,000 cases of Lyme were reported; due to questions about the reliability of blood tests and the crossover that symptoms of Lyme share with other conditions, some patient advocacy groups put this number much, much higher.[9] Fifteen years into the Lyme odyssey, Steere observed a troubling trend: patients who believed they had chronic Lyme, a persistent infection impervious to most treatments—and different from the late-term effects, such as tissue damage or inflammation, of Lyme disease.[10] He suspected that many of the patients referred to his clinic never had Lyme in the first place and likely had misdiagnosed conditions like fibromyalgia. Steere's prominence as a definitive expert on Lyme makes him all the more controversial to the patients who believe his stance on it continues to cost them their health, possibly even their lives.

On the other side are the patients and the physicians who argue that left untreated, Lyme can become a chronic condition, one that like syphilis, which shares the same spiral shape as the bacteria that cause Lyme, can result in lasting neurological damage. The parameters of the blood tests used to diagnose Lyme disease are narrow, and, as many argue, leave out certain patients who suffer from the disease. For these patients, treatment with long-term antibiotics, often intravenously, is the only option that seems to make a difference in their symptoms. Guidelines published by the Centers for Disease Control do not take into account the stories of patients whose cases went undiagnosed for too long, or cases that are complicated by co-infections, and many patients and critics feel there are worrisome conflicts of interest in funding at play among those tasked with defining these guidelines.

The medical community is by no means evenly split on the issue. Defenders of chronic Lyme who treat patients long-term are the outliers who are often under attack. Many doctors who see the need for long-term antibiotic therapy to treat Lyme disease are afraid to prescribe it for fear they will lose their licenses, since they would be going against CDC guidelines. Not only does this dispute make it difficult for patients to get diagnosed and treated, but it makes getting insurance to cover the treatment challenging, too.

"I'm lucky because I live in the most endemic area for Lyme in the country, which means that the most Lyme-literate physicians are in or around this area . . . These doctors have put their careers on the line to ensure proper treatment for their patients," Jennifer Crystal says. The phrase "Lyme-literate" is a sort of semantic carrying card to membership in the chronic Lyme population. Lyme-literate physicians are not merely educated in the various manifestations; they are recognized by patients as those who are willing to buck convention and provide long-term treatment for chronic Lyme.

College student and chronic Lyme patient Britta Bloomquist frames the debate by virtue of two poles, the Infectious Diseases Society of America and the International Lyme and Associated Diseases Society (ILADS). The IDSA wrote the original guidelines Bloomquist and many others find problematic, while the ILADS is researching and hoping to change those guidelines. Patients skeptical of the IDSA's intent in defining and treating chronic Lyme were given fodder in 2006, when Connecticut attorney general Richard Blumenthal launched an antitrust investigation into the IDSA's guideline process. He feared that conflicts of interest between the society members tasked with drafting them and the pharmaceutical and insurance companies—who had much at stake in just how narrow the treatment guidelines were—posed a significant problem. The investigation's report, issued in 2008, found serious flaws in the IDSA panel's process, including a failure to conduct conflict-of-interest reviews before appointing physicians to the panel; failure to follow its own protocols by allowing a chairman with a known bias against chronic Lyme to hand-pick panelists without scrutiny or review by an oversight committee; and failure to include physicians with dissenting views on the panel by telling them it was full, despite expanding it in later months, among other offenses.[11] A review panel put in place after the attorney general's report ultimately continued recommending against long-term antibiotic treatment, allowing insurers to deny coverage, although critics still maintain there are problems with the review process itself.

Bloomquist is no stranger to the political fallout of IDSA guidelines when it comes to treatment. In January 2010, she had taken three months of oral antibiotics to treat chronic Lyme, which had gone undiagnosed for several years. Like many patients treated for chronic Lyme, when the oral antibiotics didn't set her symptoms at bay, she had a PICC line (a peripherally inserted central catheter) inserted and did a month of IV Rocephin, one of the go-to drugs for long-term antibiotic treatment of Lyme.

"After a month, my doctor removed my PICC line because as I later found out, his hospital and clinic that he worked under was getting wary of the controversial treatment. After three days of no treatment, I could barely walk," she says. The risk of infection that PICC lines pose, as well as the potential damage to the body that high-dose, long-term antibiotics can cause, are primary reasons many physicians stand firm against this course of treatment. For the patients whose blood work does not show evidence of Lyme infection but whose clinical symptoms and narratives correspond, the risk-benefit analysis for such an intensive treatment is even steeper.

Crystal describes a similarly frustrating two-year battle to access Social Security disability benefits. The Department of Social Security didn't want to rely on her physician's reports and sent her to one of their own specialists, one who did not believe chronic Lyme existed.

"After a fifteen-minute exam in which I was hardly asked a single question about my medical history, this doctor deemed me not to have Lyme—and therefore able to work. The appeal process was a long and maddening round of getting more doctors' records and filing endless paperwork (which, ironically, I did not have the energy or mental capacity to do)," she says. She finally saw a lawyer and went before a judge who had some working knowledge of the complexity of Lyme disease and ultimately awarded her disability benefits.

"If the political controversy over Lyme didn't exist—and if more people were Lyme literate—I would not have had to fight such a ridiculous uphill battle. It's hard enough being sick; having to fight for validation, and for your rights, is like pouring salt in the wound," she says.

In *Cure Unknown: Inside the Lyme Epidemic*, veteran science writer and Lyme patient Pamela Weintraub observed that the more people she interviewed, the more obvious it became that the distance between the scientific studies and the experiences of patients was "vast." She continues,

"Peer-reviewed articles dismissing the Lyme patients' mental impairment as 'mild,' for example, did not remotely capture the experience of having a brain infection—the angst of falling behind in school or feeling perpetually foggy or confused . . . Memory loss calibrated in percentage points was presented as mere annoyance in the studies, but it translated, in patients' lives, to hours spent navigating local highways, lost in their neighborhoods, or forgetting a frying pan on the stove."[12] Weintraub's examples illustrate just how significant the subjective, lived experiences of patients are when evaluating objective measures of disease. When those experiences are multiplied over and over as they are shared on List-servs, on patient forums, and through social media sites, they become even more powerful.

It is useful to view chronic Lyme disease in the context of one of its contemporaries, chronic fatigue syndrome. Like chronic fatigue syndrome, Lyme disease first emerged in the shadow of the AIDS epidemic in the 1980s, and like chronic fatigue syndrome and fibromyalgia, it tended to appear often in middle- and upper-class Americans—in this case, those who sought refuge in leafy suburban subdivisions. Weintraub and her family entered the labyrinth of Lyme when they left New York City for the rarified green sanctuary of Chappaqua, New York, where the deer that carried the ticks responsible for Lyme were frequent visitors. In terms of gender, Lyme is more of an equal-opportunity disease than other conditions. Weintraub's own husband and two sons were eventually diagnosed with Lyme disease, but only after years of struggling in school and the workplace without a clear answer that explained their puzzling malaise.

Like the many patients with chronic fatigue and fibromyalgia around them, patients with untreated, undiagnosed Lyme are often told their complaints are mental or emotional, that if they got more rest or experienced less stress or learned to deal with their confusing array of symptoms, they just might feel better, too. Jennifer Crystal can relate. As the summer of 1997 rolled into autumn, her symptoms progressed beyond the mysterious onset of hypoglycemia. Almost immediately upon starting school, she developed flu-like symptoms. She had trouble walking and concentrating, she ran fevers, and she experienced constant muscle aches. Staff at her campus health center didn't believe her symptoms were real and began treating her as an anxious hypochondriac. One nurse even whispered that she might want to seek counseling. No one thought to look for Lyme, and routine blood tests showed nothing amiss.

"I was told that I was simply run down and stressed, maladies every college student must learn to deal with," she says.

Over the next few years, Crystal's symptoms waxed and waned. Every few months, or even weeks, she would get hit with debilitating flu-like symptoms and seemed to catch seasonal infections more often than her peers. After many trips to the hospital and the student health center, the consensus remained that she was stressed, run-down, or depressed. She doesn't dispute the stress or depression, but she insists both were a result of being so sick all the time—*not* the other way around.

After she graduated and started a teaching job in Colorado, the fluctuations continued, and more symptoms emerged: migraines, systemic hives, intense itch, shaky hands, exhaustion, racing thoughts, vivid nightmares, asthma; even her extremities burned. By age twenty-five, it was clear she could not hold down her job and she was forced to move in with her parents in her home state of Connecticut—the ground zero of the Lyme epidemic. Finally, the Lyme specialist she saw at her naturopath's suggestion listened to her entire medical history and looked at all of her symptoms as part of a whole problem, something no one had done before. Based on positive lab tests and a clinical exam, she was diagnosed with chronic persistent neurological Lyme disease, Ehrlichiosis, and Babesiosis. The last two are parasitic infections that are also transmitted through a tick bite.

"All of the strange symptoms I'd experienced over the years—from hypoglycemia to shakiness to hives to sleep disturbances—are telltale signs of one or more of these diseases. The doctor traced everything back to that day at camp in 1997. I remember a strange rash on my arm that summer—not a bull's-eye, but a series of red dots. I'd thought it was just from my sleeping bag or something . . . But looking back at it now, it seems highly probable that I was bitten by a tick that summer. My tests showed long-term and short-term exposure, which means that I may have also been reinfected at another point. Eight years later, in January 2005, I finally had my answer," she says.

Not surprisingly, the label Lyme disease bestowed to her was both a blessing and a curse.

"What some people don't understand is that many cases of Lyme, such as mine, are left undiagnosed or untreated for far too long. Over time, the spirochetes replicate and invade every system of the body. Once the bacteria enter the brain and neurological symptoms develop, it becomes next to impossible to cure someone of Lyme . . . This is why early diagnosis and treatment are absolutely critical in beating Lyme disease. I envy people who find a bull's-eye rash and get right to a doctor, because I know they will take a few weeks' worth of antibiotics and be fine," she explains.

In the end, her experiences are another reminder that differences in symptoms and diagnoses are important when it comes to treatment, but when it comes to understanding the overall implications of ongoing illness, the differences aren't nearly as striking as the similarities.

"I asked myself, what's my purpose now? How can I lead a productive life if I'm too sick to work or make contributions to society? Over time, I learned that meaningful contributions can be made even from bed (especially as a writer); that purpose goes much deeper than a job; that it's possible to create a new normal for oneself. My life isn't normal by most people's standards, but it works for me. I'm living now, not just surviving, and that's a blessing," Crystal says.

Individual Users, Collective Action: Patients and Health 2.0

Most of us have been there: we go to a doctor's office, hear a particular diagnosis, treatment, or medication, and as soon as we get a chance, we go home and look it up online. Soon, if we're lucky enough to get a diagnosis and spend some time going through the search results, we find stories of other patients whose experiences sound awfully similar to our own. Maybe we just like the comfort of knowing there are others like us out there, or maybe we locate information that we find useful in our own treatment plans or bring to discuss with our physicians. When Jennifer Crystal was finally diagnosed, she was no different. She turned to other patients living with the same diagnoses and symptoms for support, advice, and validation, and the online resources she consulted assured her that her physicians' practices were on par with those of other Lyme-literate physicians.

Doctors, nurses, and other health care professionals may still represent the first stop for people who have questions about conditions or symptoms, but research shows an increasing number of Americans turn to online resources when it comes to matters of health and wellness.[13] The Pew Research Center's Internet and American Life Project reported that 66 percent of people who report no health conditions use the Internet as a source of health information. In comparison, 51 percent of those living with chronic disease turn to the Internet for answers and information. Lack of digital access is the primary reason for the gap—not, as the report notes, lack of interest. In fact, when demographic variables are controlled, Internet users with chronic health conditions are slightly *more* likely to search online for health information than are other users.[14] Among the patients I've spoken to and connected with over years of blogging about chronic illness, I've seen lack of digital access take on many forms: some cannot afford regular access to a computer or dependable Internet. But for others, cutting through the brain fog to concentrate on online tasks is challenging, sitting upright or finding comfortable positions to type can be difficult, and working through intense pain or fatigue to focus is a regular hurdle.

Still, when they can connect, patients with chronic illness can benefit greatly from the online world. Blogging and online health discussions are especially popular avenues for people with chronic disease. Once demographic variables are controlled, being chronically ill significantly increases users' likelihood to say they work on a blog or contribute to an online discussion, a List-serv, or other online group forum that helps people with personal issues or health problems.[15] What's more, once a patient is online, living with chronic diseases is associated with a greater chance of accessing user-generated content like blog posts, hospital reviews, doctor reviews, or podcasts. This is a more dynamic use of the Internet that allows patients to use it as a means of communication, rather than simply a static source of information.[16] Patients don't just want to know the name and side effects of a medication, for example. They want to know what it is like to live with those side effects, what tips or tricks they might use to make the process easier, and if there are other treatment options that might be worth considering.

For Aviva Brandt, the journalist with the undiagnosed pain and fatigue condition, the Internet has become an essential part of her experience as a patient. As a former reporter, she is used to asking questions and needing to know all the details, so she does her own research online about everything from her myriad symptoms to the side effects of various medicines her doctor might prescribe. While the informational aspect of online resources is undeniably helpful, it is the connection and communication with other patients that has proved especially valuable.

"Blogging has saved my sanity, I think," says Brandt, whose blogging endeavors allow her to share her voice and connect with others. "It's a safe space for me to examine the progress of my mystery illness and talk about how it has affected me and my family emotionally, without feeling like I'm putting too big a burden on any one person by confiding in them . . . I hear from people who suffer similar symptoms, or love someone who does, and they share their diagnoses with me, the treatments that have been helpful and those that weren't," she says. She sees a real sense of community among those blogging on chronic health issues, and some even meet in real life.

Recent data support Brandt's online experiences. For example, Internet users with at least one chronic condition are more likely than those without to engage in the following activities: 37 percent have read someone else's health commentary online (versus 31 percent of those reporting no chronic conditions); 31 percent have watched a health video online (versus 22 percent of those reporting no chronic conditions); and 23 percent have signed up to receive e-mail updates about certain health topics, compared to 9 percent of those who do not report any health conditions.[17] Most people living with chronic illness do not attend in-person support groups and workshops—despite their utility—and instead mobilize their support system through e-mail, caregiving sites, and other social networks where they are in charge of their health narratives.[18] This makes sense, when you consider the time and physical effort it takes to make regular in-person support group meetings. Twenty percent of the users of social network sites who are living with chronic conditions use these sites to gather health information, compared with 12 percent of users of social network sites who report no chronic conditions.

"The Social Life of Health Information," a report by Susannah Fox and colleagues at the Pew Research Center's Internet and American Life Project, offers a compelling illustration of the breadth of connection and camaraderie social networks offer patients. When social network users participating in a study were asked which group was more helpful when they needed certain types of information, health care professionals were the preferred choice for technical information. However, when the questions involved how to deal with a health problem or how to find quick relief from symptoms, fellow patients, friends, and family members were favored sources.[19] The variety of resources for peer support continue to grow, from older List-servs and online discussion boards to blogs and more robust health channels and social networks such as Patients Like Me, which allows patients to share data about their conditions, symptoms, and treatments. These technologies are often lumped together under the umbrella term Health 2.0, which I use to mean networks and social media tools that allow patients (as well as health professionals) to share information. The availability of health information is important, but here the patient or Internet user as the gate-keeper of his or her health narrative is also significant.

The constant sharing and commiseration can have the opposite effect. When she was too sick to get out of bed, Jennifer Crystal joined an online support group. After a while, it became overwhelming and frustrating to read everyone else's travails, and she would end up feeling hopeless instead of hopeful. Given that my only interaction with patients with PCD is virtual—a common reality of life among people with rare diseases—I can certainly relate to Crystal's experiences. Sometimes, the e-mails that come in about treatments or doctor appointments are helpful; at other times, hearing about more deterioration, or about List-serv members joining the lung transplant list or passing away, is not what I need in that moment. For a long period of time I avoided e-mails from a celiac disease List-serv I was on because despite how many helpful, supportive posts were made, the negativity from people who were still quite angry they couldn't eat certain favorite foods was too pervasive. I was grateful I had a health condition I could actually manage without pharmaceutical intervention—something I could not claim with my other health problems—and I didn't find the anger productive.

"I have a much broader sense of what is possible and practical for a person with my illness than I might have, and this has been very important to me," Duncan Cross says. "My specific illness—Crohn's disease—is embarrassing enough that it's hard to meet people in real life who have it. Nobody really wants to talk about it with strangers. But online, we can protect ourselves with screen names and anonymity, which lets us talk more freely about our illness. And, of course, when I started blogging, I adopted a pseudonym for the same reason—so I could be more honest without worrying too much that this would end up being personally humiliating to me."

The possibilities that present themselves when patients not only have access to health information but access to each other and a vehicle through which they can organize are powerful. Cross offers an evocative analogy on this point: The interstate highway system was really important to the civil rights movement since it allowed African-Americans to move from city to city much more easily than they could on trains. That let them bring a lot of pressure to bear on specific locations, like Selma and Birmingham, in fairly short order. The highways let them act together, as a movement, in a way that was previously difficult or impossible. Now, through technology, patients separated by all sorts of boundaries—physical, cultural, emotional—are talking to each other and discussing how they can change their lives and, therefore, the world around them.

From One to Many: Virtual Patient Advocacy

We know patients use the Internet to find information and find other patients. However, the power of the Internet is more than the individual patient marshaling information and organizing caregivers and supporters. Patient advocacy, which has gained momentum since the post–World War Two era, has reached a new zenith with the advent of the Internet and Health 2.0 technologies. From Facebook and Twitter pages for disease organizations to viral campaigns and fundraising to e-newsletters to keep large numbers of patients across the country and the globe informed, mobilization that once meant sit-ins and protests now often takes place virtually. However, such mainstream accessibility also comes with a caveat: information shared online must be accurate and reliable.

It is a question we grapple with often in my science writing courses, when we debate popular versus scholarly sources or discuss why Wikipedia might serve as a resource that gives context but would not work as a scholarly source in a research paper. We probe the different purposes of writing: the personal, narrative voice that tells a story; the objective explanation of research methodology; the analytical literature review; and more. As a patient constantly tethered to my laptop, I know the importance of evaluating sources, particularly when it comes to health information. As a nonfiction writer, I know that sifting through articles and books and sourcing reference lists for other credible resources is an indispensable part of the job. I bring these experiences to bear when I tell my students that the access we have to information is an incredible opportunity, but it puts more onus on us as readers to think critically about the source, the authors, the agenda, and the validity of the information. This same analysis applies to online disease and patient advocacy groups.

"Online disease-specific groups can provide enormous support for patients in dealing with the medical and emotional chaos a chronic condition brings into their lives. It can be enormously reassuring to learn that others have had similar experiences," says Dr. Gwenn Schurgin O'Keefe, a practicing pediatrician who is actively engaged with Health 2.0 technologies.

Through her website Pediatrics Now, she maintains a regular blog and sends out e-newsletters on parenting matters and children's health. She knows firsthand the potential of the Web in terms of disseminating useful information, but she worries that people might not always give the information they find the thorough analysis it requires.

"It is much easier to get information and communicate with patients with today's Health 2.0 systems. However, patients have access to not just reliable information online but unreliable information. It is very easy for them to get misled, confused and become distrusting of health care because of the information they read online," says Dr. Gwenn, as she is referred to on the Internet. This is something that can be exacerbated when it comes to patient groups. Despite its many applications, social media can have what Dr. Gwenn calls a herd mentality, where the voice with the largest sway isn't always correctly informed.

Imagine patients in a particularly marginalized health community, like chronic Lyme or fibromyalgia, who do not feel supported or empowered by the mainstream medical community, and it is easy to see how much more influence peer commentary can have. Leah Roman, who has a master's degree in public health with a special interest in health communication and education, says people are extremely passionate about health topics and that gets magnified when patients are dealing with unknown conditions. Finding a network of support or like-minded patients who understand a patient's suffering can make an impersonal experience intimate, and out of that personal connection can come urgency and advocacy. "It's funny how that little bit of feeling included lifts spirits . . . being online does band people together, whichever side they're fighting," she says.

"I always advocate using these [online disease] sites for emotional support and to learn where to find the best care and treatments but to rely on health care professionals to get answers about medications and treatments, not empowered patients or other interested, but savvy, posters," says Dr. Gwenn. "Similarly, there is danger in these groups as the people expressing opinions are not physicians but people with opinions. It is important that people spending time on these sites realize that interpreting a person's experience with a treatment or medication is complicated and to be critical of evaluating opinions stated on these sites in light of their own experience."

It is a challenging situation, since the pull of that emotional connection and personal experience is such a gripping one. My four-year struggle with infertility, a complication of my genetic lung disease, speaks to this. While I always talked with my doctor about specific tests, medications, and results, those informational conversations only gave me part of what I was looking for: the objective, quantifiable aspects of my health status. What I really craved, and what was often much more helpful, were the experiences of other infertility patients. I wanted to hear how they dealt with loss and disappointment, how they kept going despite the doubt and sadness. I wanted to know what options they were considering, and why. It was my doctor's expertise and my own results that dictated how we approached infertility, but it was the chorus of voices I read and the collective wisdom compiled online that satisfied my emotional needs.

Like many patient communities before them, patients with Lyme disease have banded together, pushing for more coherent policies toward diagnosing and treating it, building awareness, and increasing acceptance by the mainstream medical establishment. Lyme warriors, as some are referred to, share symptoms and treatments and advocate for more recognition of their long-term illness. Groups like Time for Lyme and many others are involved in the push for more comprehensive guidelines for diagnosing and treating Lyme that are free from conflict of interest. If Kairol Rosenthal's definition of "slacktivism," where mouse clicks and link-sharing replace meaningful engagement in a cause, is one end of the advocacy spectrum, then this type of mobilization belongs decidedly at the other. The disagreement over diagnosis and treatment of chronic Lyme positions patients against individual physicians and Lyme-literate physicians against physicians who do not believe chronic Lyme exists, and it also positions the strong patient advocacy movement and all those who are caught up in it against the medical establishment itself.

New York Times reporter David Grann writes, "The rise of the Lyme disease movement—a populist torrent fueled by mass communication on the Internet as well as by cost-cutting insurance companies and bureaucratic HMO's—has become a prototype of the modern medical lobby . . . There have been lawsuits, investigations, medical suspensions, demonstrations, even death threats."[20] Patient advocacy that we've seen in decades prior tended to focus on better treatment and more research. Since conflicts of interest and dismissiveness are primary motivations for many Lyme activists, the focus of some of the most strident activism is against the medical establishment itself. Where women's health advocates saw a paternalistic, hierarchical arena, Lyme activists see a corrupt institution that cannot undertake the type of research they need. Instead, some have opted to pursue their own research. The most notable example of this is the Lyme Disease Foundation, which until it closed down in 2012, published its own journal, ran its own conferences, funded its own research, and had its own experts who weighed in with their preferred treatments.[21] Part of their success in spreading their message and garnering increased support came from the Internet—personal blogs, smaller, more local and state Lyme groups, other nonprofits, and other general-illness and advocacy sites that cross-promoted links and resources.

"I think that patient advocacy groups exist because our health care system is broken. There are many tragic stories of patients harmed by misdiagnosis, neglect, or layers of bureaucracy—and it's wonderful that they and their loved ones are fighting so that others don't share a similar fate," Dr. Val Jones says. In many ways, her observation makes sense. If the system weren't flawed, the women's health movement wouldn't have needed to upend the traditional paternalistic relationship between patient and physician. If the system weren't flawed, early HIV/AIDS activists wouldn't have had to fight so hard for the triple-drug cocktail, or people struggling with illness wouldn't have to face lack of insurance on top of their health crises. If it weren't flawed, then patients like Britta Bloomquist and so many others with Lyme disease and similarly fraught diagnoses wouldn't feel so much of their health narrative is framed within a two-sided story—us (patients and those sympathetic to their plight) versus them (the rest of the medical establishment).

However, Jones thinks that advocacy groups sometimes engage in what she describes as "misplaced passion": they mean to protect and empower others with their actions, but when they rely on false hypotheses, they can do more harm than good. She points to the autism community and the debate over the role of vaccinations in causing autism as a poignant example. Like Lyme disease, the situation surrounding autism and vaccines is a dense, complicated story, and like Lyme disease, it is the subject of many books, articles, blog posts, and impassioned arguments. The point here is not to retell that complex narrative, nor to sift through possible causes of autism. Rather, it is to look at autism within the specific context of how social media and the Internet influences patient advocacy and information sharing.

This movement is particularly intriguing since it bookends the trajectory of modern-day chronic disease: vaccinations quelled infectious diseases in post–World War Two America and paved the way for chronic diseases to emerge as significant public health and social issues. Decades later, without the looming threat of diseases like polio or smallpox, for some the pendulum has shifted. On one side are the doctors, researchers, and parents who endorse childhood vaccinations as important components of public health. On the other are those who are skeptical of the alliance between the government, the medical establishment, and the pharmaceutical companies who produce vaccines, which the skeptics believe are not made safely or dosed safely.

Nowhere is the debate about vaccines and autism as heated—and, at times, vitriolic—as online, where parenting sites, blogs, nonprofit sites, and medical and public health sites are rife with comments, opinions, and dissatisfaction. I try to imagine advocacy against vaccines and for more effective treatments for children with autism taking place in another time and context, without the immediacy and reach of social media, and it looks much different. For so many parents and advocates, the advocacy journey literally begins when they walk home from the physician's office and start researching autism online.

When parenting super-site Babble.com published an article (one of a few) by a mommy-blogger advocating against vaccinations in the summer of 2011—as well as a response to it from a pro-vaccination blogger—the comments were fast and furious, from other parents who agreed vaccination is a personal choice that belongs to each parent and doesn't affect anyone else to those who believe that matters of public health are just that—public, not personal, and the responsibility of us all.[22] Some comments were well reasoned and respectful, some were passionate, some were downright antagonistic.

My own status as a patient with compromised immune and respiratory systems places me in the highest risk category when it comes to serious manifestations and complications of infectious diseases, meaning I am on the high-priority list when it's flu vaccine time. For patients like me, the concept of herd immunity is critical. Herd immunity means that if enough of a given population is vaccinated, the likelihood of an unvaccinated person contracting that particular illness goes down. The more infectious and easily transmitted the disease, the higher the number of people who need to be vaccinated for herd immunity to work. Parents who choose not to vaccinate often rely on this built-in protection, but as more families move away from vaccinating, the protection falls apart, and those at high risk for infection because they *can't* receive vaccinations are especially vulnerable.[23]

Ginger Taylor, whose young son was diagnosed with autism, is well versed in the power of the Internet when it comes to patient advocacy. In fact, after years of researching, writing, and advocating about the association she sees between vaccines and autism, she has gone as far as forming a political party—the Canary Party—to restore a good-faith relationship between providers and patients and to rid the medical establishment of perceived corruption and conflict of interest. She also contributed a chapter to the recently published *Vaccine Epidemic: How Corporate Greed, Biased Science, and Coercive Government Threaten Our Human Rights, Our Health, and Our Children.* She is passionate about her beliefs and quick to point out that she and many advocates in the autism community are not "anti-vaccine"—the moniker often ascribed to them—but are in favor of *safer* vaccines on a safer schedule. Taylor does not agree her son even has autism but instead believes he suffered a vaccine injury that left him with encephalopathy (injury to the brain that causes symptoms similar to those of autism) that was misdiagnosed as autism. Autism isn't a medical disorder, she says, but a description of behaviors.

In an article published in *Wired* in 2009, science journalist Amy Wallace describes the backlash against vaccines as ". . . a product of the era of instant communication and easy access to information." Wallace, whose article drew intense derision from influential activists and groups who believe vaccines cause autism, continues, "The doubters and deniers are empowered by the Internet (online, nobody knows you're not a doctor) and helped by the mainstream media, which has an interest in pumping up bad science to create a 'debate' where there should be none."[24] I could practically hear the collective groan of physicians when, for example, Oprah Winfrey hosted Jenny McCarthy to talk vaccines and autism. Generation Rescue, the advocacy group espoused most famously by the actress and former *Playboy* Playmate, is often in the crosshairs of those who believe that evidence-based medicine simply does not support the association between childhood vaccinations and autism and are frustrated that social media helps spread the platform of people without medical training. McCarthy's initiation into her son's condition came via Google, where a sponsored link on a search for autism led her to the bustling community of parents and advocates who believe autism is reversible, a message her son's neurologist did not share. Like Ginger Taylor, McCarthy points out that the "anti-vaccine" tag is a misnomer: she wants a safer schedule with safe vaccines.[25]

Celebrity endorsements like McCarthy's help spread information and popularize opinions, widening the gulf between news media and conventional health communication. "Jenny McCarthy is so outspoken and has such a highly visible platform," says public health professional Leah Roman, that when she talks about her son she gives a human face to the problem, and it is difficult for science to compete with that. "There are some celebrities on the pro-vaccination campaign, but they're not being very vocal, we just don't even think of them," she says.

Physicians and public health experts would rather look at the numbers. As vaccination rates drop, cases of preventable and potentially serious infectious diseases like pertussis (whooping cough), meningitis, and measles increase. Consider pertussis, which occurred in one thousand cases in 1976 and climbed to twenty-six thousand cases in 2004 as more parents made the choice not to vaccinate.[26] Measles, declared eliminated in the United States in 2000, is on the rise in European countries and is making a comeback here, largely due to international travel. In 2008, a California boy whose parents chose not to vaccinate him caught measles while traveling in Switzerland, infecting two siblings and nine other patients, all of whom were unvaccinated.[27] That same year, the parents of ten thousand kindergarten students in California chose not to vaccinate them.[28]

That so many associate autism with vaccines is due in part to how much more we see autism now, coupled with the increase in childhood vaccinations. Today, children receive fourteen vaccines in multiple doses that total more than at any point in history, though immunologists clarify that the actual immunological challenge all those doses pose to the body is lower than in the past due to more effective vaccine development.[29] The CDC estimates that one out of every 110 children is on the autism spectrum.[30] However, since autism was first identified in the 1940s, the definition has broadened to include milder symptoms along a spectrum. That, as well as increased awareness of the symptoms and earlier detection, might help explain the prevalence.

Karen Weintraub, a health journalist and editor, has researched autism extensively for her book *The Autism Revolution*, which she wrote with Dr. Martha Herbert. She sees the autism-vaccine situation as unique from other current medical controversies in many ways. Above all, most of these advocates are parents who desperately want their once-healthy children to be better.

"They have a tremendous and crushing sense of loss. Most also feel guilty—that they could/should have protected their child from this ailment . . . it seems deeper somehow than for the parent, say, of a diabetic kid, at least among my small sampling of friends and relatives," she says. While parents whose children have other conditions may be just as likely to use social media to share information, she sees autism as an outlier because while it is fairly common, so little is known about effective treatments. Since no better explanation has emerged for what's wrong with their children, parents target vaccines.

"Shots make kids cry. Sometimes they make kids sick. Regressive autism starts around the same time as eighteen-month shots," Weintraub says, explaining why so many parents are quick to trace the onset of their children's symptoms to their vaccinations. I've spent hours reading blog posts and articles about vaccines and autism, and comment after comment from parents of children with autism starts with some variation of "my child was totally normal, healthy, and social until he/she got his/her shots." For many, that was the turning point, usually followed by unabated crying and fussiness, then stomach problems, and then the chattering and social behavior started to slow down. It is easy to look at the situation objectively and intellectually and say that correlation does not mean causation, but this drama doesn't play out in the realm of the theoretical, and that distinction means little in the face of the overwhelming emotion involved. These are parents who are scared and angry and want the best for their children.

"Frankly, the 'we must stay on message' approach of public health officials doesn't always help, either," Weintraub says, pointing out that vaccines do, in fact, harm a small number of children. The National Vaccine Injury Compensation Program was established by the federal government to pay for medical care for patients with vaccine injuries. It also relieves the liability for vaccine makers who would otherwise get out of the business. "If public health officials were or had been more willing to admit that vaccines are imperfect, the parents might have felt they'd been 'heard' by the feds, and not reacted as strongly. At this point, some public health officials will occasionally say things like this out loud, but the damage is already done."

The sense of loss, coupled with the alienation many parents feel from the medical establishment and the government, leaves a void in terms of treatment, support, and communication—and that is where technology and social media really factor. The Internet has created a class of what Ginger Taylor calls highly medically literate and informed patients and parents. Her journey began right after her young son was diagnosed. Like so many parents, she looked on a Yahoo disease group and began an online conversation with other parents whose children had the same experiences with diverse symptoms and stories—skin problems and colic as infants, noticeable changes in behavior around the time of vaccinations, gastro-intestinal difficulties, etc.—that their physicians were not taking into account or willing to discuss.

"Social media changed things dramatically," she says.

Taylor, who has a master's degree in clinical counseling and an affinity for research, jumped headfirst into the mix, collecting articles and ideas for her son's pediatrician to discuss. She read all the articles she found herself, rather than relying on the interpretation that professional societies or organizations offered. While it was helpful for her to read articles and initiate a dialogue, it strained the relationship with her son's pediatrician. The pediatrician didn't want to talk about her research and wasn't interested in discussing alternative interventions such as the gluten-free, casein-free diet many parents say helps with behavioral problems.

"For years we have heard that patients need to take more responsibility for their health and our community has," she says. She is frustrated that she is doing just that and most physicians aren't willing to collaborate with her and the many other parents out there doing the same things. It isn't just that the physicians don't want to discuss others treatments; she sees very little interest among physicians in doing the research that could actually confirm or support many of the interventions parents are already using. This unwillingness has caused a divide between parents and families and their doctors that is so pervasive many feel they have to leave mainstream medicine altogether.

"At this point, there is zero interest from people in the medical establishment in restoring faith . . . They don't care, they have their agenda, [and after] more than a decade of good-faith actions on the part of parents to work on the problem, we are met with at best being placated. At worst, they go after the doctors who help us, attack us in public, use the phrase 'desperate parent' regularly," Taylor says. "Good faith absolutely [has been] destroyed; the only thing that can change is getting corrupt public officials fired."

I asked Taylor about the charge that evidence-based medicine does not support any link between the development of autism and vaccinations.

She disagrees there is no link between vaccines and autism because she disputes the legitimacy of the evidence itself: the people who control what is published are the same ones who do the research and control the funding, and from her point of view, of course they are not going to publish research that contradicts their positions.

"It is astonishing to me how unoriginal medical corruption is," Taylor says, looking at Lyme disease and other controversial diagnoses as emerging parallels to what she and other parents and advocates have experienced, treatment she considers a "war against the patient."

Disease advocates like Taylor see the situation as a war against the patient, but many on the other side see such controversies as a war against science, with social media as a formidable force. Pro-vaccine advocates point out that vaccines give us the luxury to even think about debating them—vaccines are often called victims of their own success—and that if we lived with the immediate threat of illness or death from infectious disease previous generations did, talk of delayed vaccination schedules or opting out of vaccinations altogether would not occur.

"Of course parents are eager to discover the cause of autism so that it can be treated—but unfortunately, some have simply decided to attribute the cause to something random and unrelated. Vaccines are not the cause of autism—and some advocacy groups have squandered their energy on promoting a theory that is not based on evidence. Imagine how much more useful it would have been to direct that fervor to finding the real cause," Dr. Val Jones says. "Instead, some advocacy groups have whipped everyone into a state of paranoia over a preventive procedure (vaccination) that is one of the greatest triumphs of modern medicine." In a parallel universe, she says, scientists have discovered genes[31] associated with autism and we are now beginning to unravel the genetics of the disease. A 2011 study in *Pediatrics* found that parents who have one child with autism have a much greater risk than previously thought—a one in five chance—of having a second child with the condition. That child's risk is nearly twenty times greater than that of a child in the general population, though researchers caution that genetics alone cannot explain autism.[32]

Since it is widely believed to be a multifactorial condition, other groups are interested in exploring possible environmental and social influences further as well.

For many, the common goal—and one that is so hard to locate beneath the strife and the polarization—is more research that can answer some of these questions about what causes autism more definitively, so we can better help patients and families.

Others are concerned with making sure the scope of services offered to patients is appropriate and comprehensive, and, again, they rely on the Internet and social media to spread their message. Gina Terrasi Gallagher, a parent of a daughter with Asperger's (a high-functioning condition on the autism spectrum) and a daughter with learning disabilities, did more than participate in online conversations. She penned *Shut Up About . . . Your Perfect Kid!* a book for parents of children with special needs, and her book's social media following on Facebook numbers in the thousands and continues to grow.

"Some folks tell us that this page has saved their lives. They come here to share joys, challenges, and to exchange information. It's very difficult for folks to connect in person because they don't want to violate their children's privacy with people who know them. The Facebook page allows them to connect with parents around the world who 'get it.' Many parents have suffered in silence with no one to talk to. Now when something happens, they have a place to share their news or vent," she says.

Gallagher knew she had to be cautious about looking up information for her daughter online. With the abundance of interventions and advice out there, it is difficult to wade through and figure out what is legitimate, especially when parents feel they can't turn to their children's pediatricians for help.

"I think it's critical that pediatricians have this knowledge and provide compassion to parents. It's overwhelming to learn your child has a disability and difficult to know where to turn since there is so much information out there online," she says.

Still, the benefits are clear. For Gallagher, social media has presented opportunities not just for emotional support or connection but for education and advocacy as well. Her advocacy is focused on helping her daughters get the most support and resources they need to meet with the most success. She is less concerned with sourcing why her daughter manifested autism (though she does think there is something to the vaccination link), particularly since her daughter is doing so well.

"I'm sure if she were struggling, I would be more outraged and committed to finding a cure and finding the source of the disability," she says. "My daughter hates when people talk about 'curing her.' It makes her sound as though she is not okay the way she is. I've tried to tell her that she's a bright person capable of achieving all the goals she sets in life." In that sense, Gallagher is making the same choice parents, patients, advocates, and organizations across the disease spectrum must make, and have been making for decades: where best to allocate our time, energy, and resources.

How did we get from Jennifer Crystal, one patient dealing with the lifelong effects of a tiny tick bite, to Aviva Brandt's assertion that blogging saved her sanity, all the way to the online debates over vaccines and autism? Patients became wired, and as individuals, logging onto their computers became something much more than locating definitions or looking up symptoms. It became the antidote to the alienation, isolation, and skepticism so many felt. Technology amplified our questions and our worries, our assumptions and our expectations. Without question, chronic Lyme and autism are richly detailed and harrowing case studies in present-day disease and advocacy. However, in the broader context of chronic illness and technology, they illustrate a new twist in the "us versus them" mentality, one that goes beyond the usual divisions. This new chasm is one that social media make possible: the old guard of conventional medicine, rooted in medical journals and conferences, versus the new guard, who use everything from Twitter and Facebook to blogs, podcasts, and viral petitions and campaigns to share information and collaborate.

The immediacy of social media, where links go out in real time and off-the-cuff remarks have a permanent Internet footprint, is a central factor here. Dissemination of information works much differently in the public health sphere, and in research in general. It can take several years for a

study to come together, and even longer for it to go through the peer review process and eventually get published in a journal. "Public health officials are trained not to make statements without research to back it up,"
says Leah Roman. When it comes to social media, "[this] doesn't work to
our advantage."

The Internet and social media platforms are the direction advocacy is
headed, which signals that like it or not, evidence-based medicine is going
to need to utilize these same technological capabilities on an even greater
scale. If my personal Twitter feed is any indication, hospitals, research organizations, and public health entities have a more visible online presence
than even a couple years ago, and the availability of published research
online and prepublication previews certainly adds immediacy to the long,
behind-the-scenes process involved in academic and research publishing.
Roman agrees, adding that some public health programs have health communications tracks and there is a growing effort in training practitioners to
do more qualitative research, interviews, and focus groups to widen their
skill sets. All the traditional rules of effective health communication, such
as professional, tailored writing that addresses its audience appropriately,
still apply when we use social media.

"I always advise health care providers to be part of the conversation
so I do think it would help evidence-based medicine to utilize social media
more to help combat the myths out there for vaccines, autism and so many
other issues in the health care industry," says Jones. Her website getbet
terhealth.com added weekly content features from the CDC in 2011, citing
a shared goal of reaching as many people as possible and providing them
with scientifically accurate information.

I can see why Ginger Taylor and the parents and laypeople advocating for what they consider a safer vaccine schedule feel the situation is a
"war against patients": they feel dismissed, even deceived, by the medical
establishment that is meant to help their children. There are many cre-
vasses that are likely too wide for the sides to meet, especially when it
comes to accepting the conclusions of evidence-based medicine as au-
thoritative and legitimate or not. However, I can't help but wonder if the
divisions wouldn't be so dramatic and the social media fallout so conten-

tious if, in those initial encounters in exam rooms and hospitals, in those first exchanges of Internet research and queries, patients and parents felt more supported, and physicians felt less besieged. The ingredient that seems to be missing so often is collaboration. It is a new iteration of an all-too-familiar problem. When I consider the Tired Girls, those living in chronic pain, or those living with rare or hard-to-diagnose diseases, the absence—or at the very least, the *perceived* absence—of collaboration lays claim there, too.

I mentioned a pendulum swing in terms of parental attitudes toward vaccination, but both examples in this chapter illustrate a broader shift, too. In mid-twentieth-century America, science represented the great savior. Vaccines could prevent the scourge of infectious disease, antibiotics could fend off harmful bacteria, and we felt we had more control over disease and therefore our destinies. By the end of the twentieth century and the first decade of the twenty-first, the science itself came under fire. Our misstep back then was, if anything, an arrogance that elevated the reach of science. Now, even as patients yearn for biological evidence of disease for validation and accommodation, it is not always seen as a sacrosanct seal of proof.

CHAPTER 8

Participatory Medicine and Transparency

W HEN Dave deBronkart was told he had a rare, late-stage kidney cancer in 2007, his diagnosis had a median survival time of just twenty-four weeks. DeBronkart took to the Internet, scouring research on treatments and connecting with other patients to see how he could survive what was considered an unbeatable disease. Armed with research and a wealth of information from other patients, he brought his results to his treating physician, and together, they came up with a plan.

He was engaging in what researcher Susannah Fox describes as a "revolution in health care [that] is running along a parallel track, mixing people's instincts to share knowledge with the social media that make it easy, creating what might be called 'peer-to-peer healthcare.'"[1] Data suggests this peer connection is especially useful for patients with rare diseases. Survey results revealed that those living with rare disease, their own or a loved one's, have developed keen researching skills to both cope with and minimize the challenges and setbacks associated with rare diseases, forming a "collective pursuit taken on by bands of brothers- and sisters-in-arms who may never meet up in person."[2]

With the support and engagement of his physician, deBronkart used the results of his intensive research and peer feedback in his treatment plan, participated in a clinical trial, and, against overwhelming odds, survived the rare and lethal disease. Clinical trials themselves are an extension of this revolution in health care: technology and social media now play an important role in making participation in trials accessible and possible, and at-home monitoring and electronic data collection make studies on diseases with large patient bases more feasible. These networks are also a natural place to recruit patients and promote ongoing trials.

DeBronkart is now a frequent speaker as e-Patient Dave at health care conferences around the world; he is an active and respected blogger, and he published his first book, *Laugh, Sing, and Eat Like a Pig: How an Empowered Patient Beat Stage IV Cancer (and What Healthcare Can Learn from It)*, in 2010. His experiences embody the spirit of e-patients, those who are "empowered, engaged, equipped, and enabled."[3] He and his colleagues who write and think about participatory medicine want patients to have health care information available and transparent to them—their own health information as well as the research and data that exists virtually. A permanent, portable electronic record of patient health information benefits providers and patients alike and supports collaboration and empowerment. Despite the inherent risks of data breaches and privacy concerns that are inevitable when we shift information online, the adoption of electronic health records is a big—and necessary—part of the evolution of participatory medicine.

For those with chronic disease, this idea of transparency extends to all facets of their lives as patients. Dr. Kevin Pho, a primary care physician, writes at KevinMD.com, where his popularity has earned him the accolade "the Web's most influential health care social media platform."[4] As a blogger and contributor to *USA Today*, the *New York Times*, and other national outlets, Pho is well positioned to evaluate the influence technology has on the health care system and its users. The past ten to fifteen years have done a lot for patient empowerment in terms of giving patients access to information, though such access raises issues. For example, he mentions that only about a quarter of patients who consult the Internet or print out health information check the sources of that information, so a person or company trying to sell something has potentially as much influence as a reputable source like a hospital or public health organization. The problem is, it isn't always easy for patients to tell the difference, and, as Pho points out, it isn't always a priority for the patient to discern that difference.

"Most doctors and patients are navigating through it and need to proceed cautiously and doctors need to realize the paradigm of the empowered patient," Pho says. Examples like the e-patient movement "show what potential patients have when they have info and can play an active role," he says. It is up to doctors not only to accept the empowered patient but to embrace that type of patient. The longer it takes doctors to do this, the wider the distance grows between patient and provider.

Participatory medicine holds the premise that technology can fundamentally benefit patients and the doctor-patient relationship, and when used appropriately, that information can be the bridge that connects both parties. In a white paper the late Dr. Tom Ferguson was drafting with the "e-Patient Scholars Working Group," he wrote, "Something akin to a system upgrade in our thinking is needed—a new cultural operating system for healthcare in which e-patients can be recognized as a valuable new type of renewable resource."[5] I appreciate this notion of a renewable resource, of the patient as someone with inherent value that remains and extends beyond an interaction. This could mean taking care of their own disease management, helping or supporting other patients, or participating in clinical trials the way deBronkart did.

Participatory medicine is an inherent extension of what David B. Morris wrote about postmodern illness—how the ways we live and work have shifted from the industrial to the technological, and how that factors in the experience of illness. Narratives take place virtually now, not just in physical spaces of exam rooms and hospital beds, and the conversation is changing because we have different tools at our disposal. The challenge remains how to use those tools most effectively, especially when there is so much information that threatens to distract or misguide us.

"Culture lives in conversations between people, what they say is possible and not possible . . . we out here on the leading edge can see that vision that healthcare is about engaging patients, but meanwhile the street reality is where people are not treated well," deBronkart says. "It is natural when culture is changing for people to get it wrong at first. We start out naïve when something new becomes possible. We gain experience, discover what works, and correct ourselves . . . When you start talking about something new, people who hear it hear it in their current view of the world." For many, this context used to be that physicians know everything, patients know nothing, and patients were lucky to even get time with their physician. Culture change is not easy, seamless, or immediate on either side, and simply barging into a physician's life with e-mail or downloaded information is not an appropriate way to bring about culture change.

A now famous 2007 *Time* magazine article, "When the Patient Is a Googler," tells the story of a surgeon "punting" a patient to a colleague after being subject to a monologue filled with misinformation and apparent self-absorption. Dr. Scott Haig writes, "Every doctor knows patients like this. They're called 'brainsuckers.' By the time they come in, they've visited many other docs already—somehow unable to stick with any of them. They have many complaints, which rarely translate to hard findings on any objective tests. They talk a lot."[6] Haig has no problem with patients researching health conditions beforehand; rather, he contends it was the patient's attitude—too aggressive, perhaps; too confident in medical hypotheses—that was a roadblock in their relationship.

In 2011, *Time* ran another article about patients who google health information, but by this point, there was a noticeable shift in perspective. Here, Dr. Zachary F. Meisel opines that it is not productive to debate the practice of searching for health information, since, as we know, searching is so common. Instead, health professionals should ask themselves what they can do to help the process and thereby help their patients achieve better health. The keys are engaging patients in shared decision making, providing them with credible, peer-reviewed health resources, and acknowledging that patients are doing right by getting informed.

Not every patient who comes in with a stack of printouts is a cyberchondriac, and not every physician who gets frustrated with misinformation is unreceptive to patients' research. How do we avoid falling into the trap of these extremes? DeBronkart describes the process as more of an awakening.

"The number one thing is ongoing culture change so that clinicians learn it can be valuable and legitimate; the other side is patients learning how to google more effectively so that what they bring in is less likely to be junk . . . as we move forward with this social change, ideally patients will learn to be smarter about their research . . . [with] physicians learning how to coach them," he says. For example, his primary care physician will ask patients during interviews what kind of information they look at online. When deBronkart finds something new he takes it in and asks what his physician thinks about it, rather than framing it as an indictment that the doctor is negligent or uninformed if he has been doing or not doing a particular thing. His physician might agree, might say avoid the treatment, or might say he is not sure, and they will talk about further strategy.

The ideas of responsibility and transparency so ingrained in participatory medicine have a far reach: researching and participating in alternative treatments; the direct-to-consumer advertising of pharmaceuticals and the challenges that poses to the doctor-patient relationship; the lifestyle decisions and behaviors that can lead to or cause progression in certain chronic conditions. The patient advocacy movements we looked at in the previous chapter were ones that, however inevitably, often ended up working against the medical establishment. Participatory medicine is a model for moving forward *within* the medical establishment as empowered patients—and the very tools that make this change possible are the same ones that can distract from this forward motion.

Options and Agendas: Making Choices in the Digital Age

The term "patient" itself is as nuanced and revealing as the distinctions we make between terms like "illness," "disease," "sickness," or "disability." The term "patient" can connote passivity, and not just because of its association with the personal characteristic of *being* patient. Some argue patients are essentially consumers and that health care is an economic transaction. While that is true, the complexity of health care is not captured adequately if we discuss it entirely in business terms. Fred Trotter, a

blogger, information technology specialist, and advocate for patients accessing their health information, points out that information parity makes
the patient-as-consumer angle problematic.[7] While the move toward more
transparency in reporting safety, errors, costs, and other criteria has momentum, when we want more information on, say, a procedure or surgery
at a hospital, we have much less immediate and comprehensive data than
we would if we were looking to purchase an automobile.

Trotter's point resonates. As a first-time mother, I thoroughly researched
baby gear, trends, and safety issues. We even had the latest baby-gear issue of *Consumer Reports* (itself a gift) with us when we registered, only
pulling out car seats and high chairs with the highest safety and consumer satisfaction ratings. Yet I had very little data in terms of comparing hospitals or intervention outcomes. Likely I could have gotten at least
some of this information, but I didn't try. Part of it was the belief, right or
wrong, that my world-renowned hospital with its equally world renowned
neonatal intensive care unit (NICU) and its roster of Harvard-educated
specialists and subspecialists represented the best care possible. Part of it
was that my own particular pregnancy had a set of risks and variables that
most others didn't because of my rare diseases, so I began to feel like the
basic obstetrics numbers didn't really apply to me—after all, they really
hadn't up until that point.

What I did have was a considerable amount of information on the
risks and potential outcomes of prematurity at every stage from viability
through late-term prematurity, and copious information on side effects
and contraindications of all the medicines that could possibly be used to
treat me during my pregnancy. I had developed many scenarios of how a
pregnancy could implicate my health conditions, and vice versa. I had the
experiences of a couple of women with PCD who'd been pregnant, and
the experiences my specialist had treating one pregnant patient with PCD.
I had constant data on the baby's progress and on my own health status,
information gleaned from weekly tests that we used to make decisions at
each stage of the pregnancy. I now realize just how much of my pregnancy
and our mutual outcomes depended on both collaboration and availability
of information. Emotionally, I always felt the presence of this stream of

data about our baby and its ability to reassure me, frighten me, or paralyze me, mid-decision. But from an intellectual standpoint, I see how intricately information and survival are linked.

While patients often have expertise in their own bodies and symptoms, being a "patient expert," another term under scrutiny, certainly does not imply that physicians and patients have the *same* expertise and knowledge, making the role of the physician obsolete.[8] But a patient with chronic disease often has to play several roles—we *do* make comparisons and make choices, we *are* expected to be patient, we *are* experts in our own manifestations of disease, and, more than ever, we need to be informed collaborators in our health care experience.

People with chronic illness are avid consumers of information and products and services, and represent a source of ongoing and often escalating needs. Our weak point, though, stems from precisely this need for continual treatment: the siren's song of a cure, a seductive phenomenon for patients with chronic illness. We must continuously navigate between hope and optimism, acceptance and adaptation. If we focus exclusively on the promise of a cure, we risk losing sight of what we need to do in the present to best manage our health. If we never indulge in the hope for a cure, we risk burnout, resentment, possibly even despair. Accepting the present reality of our health conditions doesn't mean giving up on the idea of hope, but acceptance shouldn't mean we don't look for ways to improve our situations, either.

I follow type 1 diabetes bloggers who are on the receiving end of frustrating pitches promising to "cure" their disease, though anyone with credible knowledge of type 1 diabetes knows it is an autoimmune disease in which the pancreas no longer works, meaning patients are dependent on insulin—which is by no means a cure. I regularly get unsolicited pitches claiming a particular expert's regimen will help me, or this particular homeopathic concoction will make breathing easier. I skim, delete, and shake my head. A cure is not something I think about all that much; I'm focused on living the best life I can with the constellation of problems I have. However, I know that the potential of a cure lives in a laboratory, not in some unsophisticated PR flack's pitch. The onus is on me to know when to pay attention and when to shuffle such items to my mental spam box. The most serious condition I have is a genetic one, so until someone figures out how to grow cilia in a lab, I don't put much stock in such entreaties.

"It's really hard to accept the limits of modern medicine," observes Dr. Val Jones. "We can't cure every disease, we can't effectively treat every symptom, and we can't prevent death indefinitely. It's human nature to want to control our destinies, to reject the cards we've been dealt. In that sense I have the utmost sympathy for people who choose to turn over every treatment stone in the face of a daunting diagnosis, or when they are suffering from disease." However, when we are sick we are at our most vulnerable, and she sees companies preying on that vulnerability by offering false hope—often in the form of expensive treatments. "They know that we'll do anything when we're suffering, including buying into a carefully constructed fantasy (often couched in 'medical-sounding' jargon). Peddling fake medicine to sick people is morally unjustifiable," she says. Opportunists have always been around; now, their presence is that much more intrusive—they're in our in-boxes, they pop up in our Web browsers, and they approach us in sympathetic ways. It's easy to spot the true charlatans, those peddling the gimmicks. More complex issues arise for patients and providers when it's a difference of evidence and interpretation, not some fraudulent scam, and this is where the idea of informed choice really factors.

It's all about the validity of the information, Barbara Kivowitz reminds us. When a patient is newly diagnosed, desperate or scared, or has exhausted all treatment options without finding relief, she admits, it is very easy to be swayed by personality, rather than by accuracy. "As much as we search for answers, we have to accept that the sands are always shifting and what we are doing and what we are told today might be different five years from now . . . [The] seeker needs to put quotation marks around the truth and keep seeking and be one's own research validator and see what repeats and what appears to be credible based on common sense," she says. When her pain was out of control, she fell susceptible to the claims of a doctor she found online who said his approach worked, and that the only reason the medical community didn't accept it was because it cost so much less. As her regular physician pointed out, wouldn't other professionals know about it and do research if this person really had found a cure? She learned a valuable lesson about the importance of aggregating sources and looking at the issue through multiple lenses. In her case, this included conventional medicine, trusted medical sources, as well as complementary and alternative medicine.

For patients with chronic illness, complementary and alternative medicine (CAM) is a particularly relevant example of the competition between what we want from medicine and what the evidence at hand can give us in terms of informed choice. CAM is a set of diverse practices and treatments that are grouped into broad categories that include natural products like herbal supplements; mind-body practices like meditation, acupuncture, and yoga; body manipulation and body-based practices like massage; and energy-based practices like reiki, which is a therapeutic touch technique. For millions of Americans, especially those living with chronic pain, CAM is a popular choice and has made a difference in quality of life. Some patients count their physicians as supportive of their choice to practice CAM, even if so far the science does not support its safety or effectiveness. For others, it's not something they are willing to disclose to their physician, eliminating the opportunity for collaboration. It is undoubtedly a lucrative business; each year, Americans spend nearly $21 billion in nutritional supplements alone.[9]

Janet Geddis, the woman living with debilitating migraines, practices CAM and makes conscious diet and lifestyle choices that are a regular part of her disease maintenance. She takes daily supplements and practices yoga, tai chi, and mindful meditation. Her complementary care physician recommended a smoothie recipe customized for her particular health needs that she makes every day, and she tries to incorporate regular exercise, like walking, several times a week. She has "dabbled" in CAM for a long time, but has been a devotee for two and a half years. She needs and uses her conventional Western treatments to help when she senses a migraine is imminent—specifically, a triptan drug, designed to help abort migraine attacks—but her supplements, smoothies, and activities help keep her whole system in equilibrium, which she says leads to fewer migraine attacks and pain flare-ups. When the triptans have done their best but the migraines still grab hold of her and won't let go, she has rescue medicines (narcotics) that help with the pain but don't necessarily do much for the debilitating side effects, such as dizziness, nausea, and photophobia.

In December 2008, the National Center for Complementary and Alternative Medicine (NCCAM) and the National Center for Health Statistics (part of the Centers for Disease Control and Prevention) released findings on Americans' use of CAM. The data suggests that experiences like Geddis's and of many other patients living with chronic pain and illness are more common than one might think. For example, in 2007, nearly four out of ten American adults (38 percent) reported having used some form of CAM in the previous twelve months. The CAM therapies they had most commonly used were non-vitamin and non-mineral natural products such as fish oil, glucosamine, flaxseed oil, and ginseng; deep breathing exercises; meditation; chiropractic or osteopathic manipulation; massage; and yoga.[10] CAM use as detailed in the 2007 survey was more prevalent among women, adults aged thirty to sixty-nine, adults with higher levels of education, adults who were not poor, former smokers, and adults who had been hospitalized in the previous year. Of note, the period between 2002 and 2007 also saw numerous positive articles about CAM in the popular press, as well as an increase in the number of licensed practitioners. As such, more awareness coupled with more opportunity may help explain the growing popularity of CAM.[11]

Do I think acupuncture, reiki, or other practices will conjure up working cilia for me? Obviously not. Do I think they can cure what ails patients with chronic conditions? No, but I don't think that's the expectation most people have when they try CAM. Usually, they are trying to help treat their symptoms—their pain, inflammation, or fatigue, for example— not cure the precipitating condition altogether. In fact, research shows that in 2007, the most common conditions people used CAM to help treat included back pain, head/chest colds, neck and joint pain, arthritis, and anxiety/depression.[12] There are boundaries to what science can do in terms of understanding, treating, and eliminating pain, and the "complementary" aspect of CAM refers to those patients who use it in conjunction with conventional treatment, such as prescription drugs. Often, it's when those drugs have reached the end of their usefulness that patients seek out treatments that are beyond the pale of Western medicine.

Roy Porter contends that this upswing in CAM shows that regular medicine is no longer convincing in its role as the best means to cure patients, and that promises made about lethal diseases and the numerous intractable chronic conditions we live with have not been delivered. In the post–World War Two era of irresistible progress, people began to expect that we were just a breath away from conquering so much of what ailed us. We've lost that naïveté and that arrogance, and, in some instances, perhaps at the expense of our trust in the medical establishment. What's more, we live in a society that increasingly values choice and self-assertiveness, which translates into how we approach medical problems. Porter writes, "Affluence, education, leisure and any of the values promoted by corporate capitalism have stoked a culture of individual enhancement and free and active choice. As with cars, careers or sexual partners, it has become the done thing to shop around for healing—whether in desperation, as an exercise of the power of the purse, or as part of an odyssey of life."[13]

An integrative model of health, in which the mind, body, spirit, and even community are key components of health, is indeed popular in today's wellness lexicon. The focus is on treating the whole person, rather than managing symptoms, and in that respect, it is both progressive as well as a throwback to more ancient notions of healing. The growing popularity of mind-body practices is a testament to the fact that for many patients, the biomedical model of illness upon which conventional medicine relies comes up short. Top research hospitals and institutions are starting to operate mind-body and CAM clinics, and under the auspices of the National Institutes of Health, NCCAM is the federal government's primary agency dedicated to researching practices beyond the scope of conventional medicine.[14] Since 1999, the number of medical schools that have joined the Consortium of Academic Health Centers for Integrative Medicine, an organization that helps schools incorporate education on CAM, has risen from eight to fifty.[15]

While the NCCAM may give legitimacy and validation to those who believe CAM works and are hopeful the science will soon follow to prove this, that position is not uniformly accepted. Proponents of evidence-based medicine have taken to blogs and online media to echo their concerns. Writing for Science-Based Medicine, Dr. Steven Novella contends that the CAM and integrative labels are at once both marketing attempts to re-brand as medicine what fails to meet the usual criteria for it, as well as more damaging attempts to create a separate standard of scientific re-search. He writes, "People who are being studied tend to take better care of themselves and are more compliant with treatments (because they are being watched). They may also feel better as a result of the positive atten-tion from a health care provider—old-fashioned good bedside manner. These are some of the variables being controlled for. But it is scientifically absurd to argue that they justify an ineffective treatment. But that is ex-actly what CAM proponents are doing."[16]

Against this backdrop, it is not surprising to see that 61 percent of Americans don't feel they can discuss their use of CAM with their physi-cians, and the majority of physicians don't inquire about supplements or CAM practices their patients might be using.[17] On many levels, this dis-tance is damaging. For one, patients face potential risk of drug interac-tions, but it is the quality and integrity of the relationship itself that suffers when patients feel they cannot be open and physicians are not aware of this whole other aspect of patients' lives.

The distinction is not about degrees with evidence-based medicine— it is about the science. Out of forty systematic reviews of acupuncture, massage, naturopathy, and yoga published between 2002 and 2007 in PubMed, the National Library of Medicine's research database, ten arti-cles (25 percent) found sufficient evidence to conclude that a specific CAM therapy was effective in treating a specific condition. Acupuncture and yoga were found to help back pain, and acupuncture was effective for patients with knee pain, insomnia, and nausea/vomiting (and that includes patients who were postoperative, receiving chemotherapy, or were pregnant).[18]

"So the bottom line is this: wanting to fight against disease is a good thing. But the most important battles are won with science. Compassion and kindness are part of good medical care—and CAM is usually no more than an expensive distraction from real cures or acceptance of our physical situations," Dr. Jones says.

Despite that, patients continue to choose CAM and find positives in it. Part of what makes Janet Geddis's mind-body integration so productive is that both her CAM practitioner and her primary care physician are knowledgeable and supportive of the other's perspective—there is no "us versus them" mentality in a collaborative situation like this.

"One thing that surprised me most about my CAM health care provider was how he isn't judgmental at all regarding so-called 'Western' medicine. He recognizes that my prescription triptan drugs help me cope with migraine attacks and has never asked me to go off my prescription medications. He has a fairly strong knowledge of so-called traditional medicinal approaches and doesn't tend to frown upon them, as I'd expected," she says. "My primary care physician is, to my happiness, really supportive of the care I receive from the hospital's Mind-Body Institute and is good at making sure that her recommendations complement my CAM doctor's recommendations. Having doctors respect each other—even if they only know of each other through me—makes things so much smoother."

Remember too that for many patients, the decision to try out CAM techniques comes after a long, frustrating trial-and-error existence within the confines of conventional medicine. When nothing else has worked, there is much less to risk losing, especially when relief is nowhere to be found. That is why CAM is so appealing to the millions of people living with constant pain and ongoing symptoms. Those who have implemented some type of alternative treatment usually aren't trying to buck the conventional medical system or take a stand against evidence-based medicine. They aren't trying to make an ideological point, they aren't trying to be contrary, difficult, or any other characteristics that might be lobbed at them from those who doubt the value of CAM. They want to feel better, and they will exhaust every option available to them in search of that relief.

Barbara Kivowitz uses a combination of CAM methods to help manage her chronic pain. She feels the advent of CAM's popularity is symptomatic of a larger social and political question: Should medicine be strictly evidence-based or designer medicine for individual patients? For patients with complex chronic conditions, the notion that every case is really a case of one is that much more relevant. Obviously the medical establishment and the research it conducts rely on the integrity of evidence-based medicine, as do so many patients with disease, particularly clear-cut ones. But for those for whom the evidence-based treatments are not working, and for those whose problems stretch beyond what we can identify, looking outside of what is conventional is often born out of necessity. The battle over science will continue, but for now patients who make the informed decision to implement CAM and the physicians who manage their conditions share a burden of disclosure and communication. In that way, CAM is but the latest iteration of a much larger pattern of responsibility and decision making.

We are at an interesting crossroads. We know more about disease than ever before and as patients, we have access to more health information than at any point in human history. At the same time, there are so many competing agendas that threaten to get in the way of collaboration. The progress that has given us fewer invasive surgeries, more accurate diagnostic tests and refined therapies, and protection against communicable disease has raised our expectations. In *Better than Well*, Carl Elliott observes that we turn to and depend on technology to fix our inconveniences and dissatisfactions, even if it isn't always the appropriate solution.[19] While we profess to enjoy competitive sports, Elliott considers, it is important that we win the game, so performance-enhancing drugs become more popular. We want to look good so others will both notice and emulate us, so the use of cosmetic surgery and other enhancement techniques increases. Thanks to technology, many of us have become accustomed to immediate answers and results, and often we expect our bodies and the care and management of them to follow suit. Chronic illness—its lingering symptoms, its diagnostic subterfuges, its frequent defiance of data and easy answers—challenges this worldview. Not only that, it sometimes removes us from the competition altogether.

So are we better or worse off for the resources we have at our disposal? For patients like me who likely wouldn't be alive or would have significantly shorter life spans and more suffering without technology, at the most basic level, it's not a question that merits too much consideration. Survival wins. But if we move past fundamental issues of mortality and morbidity, when we ask ourselves whether all the resources we have within reach actually bring us more relief, satisfaction, or qualitatively better interactions and communications, the answer isn't so black and white.

"I think we like to mythologize previous generations, as if they were somehow better—tougher, perhaps—for not having had various technologies and treatments available. I can think of maybe a few instances, but in general I think this is greatly overstated," says Duncan Cross. As an example he uses depression, a condition that typically went untreated in previous generations. "Now we have lots of pills that we can take, and to some extent this has encouraged us to view as pathologies what are in fact some very normal moods and feelings. But the fact is, previous generations were no better off for untreated depression. I know that in my family, there were a few people who were probably exactly that—depressed and untreated. They might have been tougher at some level, but they weren't better people for being untreated," he says.

Cross mentions depression for good reason. One out of every ten Americans takes an antidepressant, and we have seen a doubling of patients seeking prescription medication for depression between 1996 and 2005.[20] The numbers are a revealing look into the cultural mood we find ourselves in. In an essay for *Salon*, Charles Barber, a lecturer in psychiatry at Yale, says that right now, there is "a high-water mark of worry and suffering on numerous fronts—economic, of course, but also social, with our ever-increasing isolation and Internet-driven loss of human connection and the ongoing trauma of wars and crises that just don't seem to end."[21] Part of the reason is what Barber mentions—economic stress, alienation, feeling disconnected from each other and from our physicians. But part of the reason is that in the midst of our fears and vulnerabilities we are inundated with persuasive advertisements for a whole host of drugs, including many for depression, anxiety, and other mental health conditions.

One of the most obvious marks of the consumer society in which we live is not simply the abundance of prescription drugs, but the direct-to-consumer (DTC) advertising of them. They are almost exclusively targeted toward people with chronic health conditions. Think about how many heart patients take cholesterol-lowering statins, how many asthmatics rely on inhalers for daily maintenance and rescue situations, or how many watery-eyed allergic adults reach for antihistamines and nasal spray. Consider how much money that translates into for the companies that produce these medicines. We spend a whopping $250 billion annually on prescription drugs. They are the fastest growing medical expenditure, and it is not just because more people are taking prescriptions. The drugs we take are more likely to be newer and more expensive—the same ones we see on television and splashed across magazines—than older, cheaper (but otherwise effective) drugs, and the prices of many heavily prescribed drugs are frequently raised.[22] Not coincidentally, total spending on pharmaceutical promotion grew from $11.4 billion in 1996 (when DTC advertising became legal) to $29.9 billion in 2005. During that time, spending on DTC advertising increased by 330 percent, making up 14 percent of total promotional expenditures in 2005.[23]

Barber observes that the commodification of pharmaceuticals, right alongside cars, household goods, and other products, is "a very American thing," something a whole generation has grown accustomed to seeing.[24] In fact, America is the only country other than New Zealand that allows DTC advertising. There is an entire generation of potential patients who have grown up seeing drug ads and don't remember things any other way. I know this firsthand, because I meet members of this generation every semester when I greet my new health sciences students. This self-selected group is more aware of the ads than other majors might be, particularly the pharmacy students, but for people their age, drug ads are simply a part of daily life. It is hard to flip through a magazine or sit through a television program without seeing an ad for a new prescription drug. From the "purple pill" campaign (Nexium) to the fluttering nighttime Luna moth (Lunesta) to the ubiquitous buzzing bees, insects, and wind-tousled flowers that dominate commercials for allergy medications, the DTC marketing of pharmaceutical drugs has dramatically altered the way patients and physician interact and has challenged the basic notion of what constitutes an illness. With celebrities endorsing drugs to grow longer eyelashes or relieve restless leg syndrome now firmly entrenched in the popular consumer health lexicon, critics of DTC advertising charge that drug companies are "creating" diseases so patients will see themselves in the ads and ask their physicians for a prescription.

One such critic is Jennifer Shaw. For over eight years, Shaw was a top-ranking sales representative for Big Pharma, until she left the industry to write her memoir, *Big Pharma's Sexy Little Secret*, detailing the behind-the-scenes machinations of the pharmaceutical sales industry.

"Many patients are walking into their doctor's office demanding specific medications that they saw on TV . . . Once the patient feels they need to be on that specific medication, there is little a doctor can do to persuade them otherwise. Anything else the doctor puts the patient on will now 'not work.' The patient is basically brainwashed from the DTC [advertising]," Shaw says.

Brainwashed, possibly—unless, of course, that patient approaches his or her doctor with questions about the medication, about the symptoms he or she is experiencing that resonate with the ad, and they have a conversation about it. That's the ideal situation worth striving for, but the issue is, how do we ensure that happens?

In the fifteen years it has been legal, skeptics have had concerns over the safety of the drugs that are featured in DTC advertising, mainly through television ads. Also at issue is the Food and Drug Administration's ability to enforce regulations that ads must accurately reflect the balance of a drug's benefits and risks. Research published in the *New England Journal of Medicine* found that while we know spending on DTC advertising increased 330 percent between 1996 and 2005, the number of letters sent to companies from the FDA indicating violations of these regulations dropped from 142 in 1997 to 21 in 2006.[25] It turns out that drug companies fare dismally when it comes to properly advertising prescriptions to health care professionals (the one writing the scripts), too: a study published in 2011 found that of 192 pharmaceutical ads published in biomedical journals, a mere 18 percent were fully compliant with FDA guidelines. More than half (58 percent) of the ads failed to quantify serious risks, while 48 percent lacked verifiable references.[26] Researchers attribute this lack of oversight and compliance to inadequate resources at the FDA, and hope that updating FDA guidelines to include more transparency, particularly with safety and efficacy information, will improve the quality of information given to physicians.[27]

Pharmaceutical companies and other proponents of DTC advertising contend that it exists to give patients and physicians educational information about various conditions and treatment options. It is a form of patient education, and readily available patient education is a positive development and a tool for collaboration. However, a major complaint about DTC ads is that TV commercials fail to adequately portray the serious risks of prescription drugs. Factors such as the speed at which side effects are mentioned, the rapid pace at which images flicker on the screen, and the feel-good quality of those images (fields of flowers and butterflies, families cavorting on the beach or in a park) can distort the impact of a drug's serious risks. It is unclear whether patients are well enough versed to weed through the distractions—or, more pertinently, whether they are even given ample opportunity to do so. FDA laws require a "fair balance" of information, meaning that the content and delivery of a drug's primary risks must be presented in a similar way to its primary benefits.[28] This does not mean benefits and risks warrant equal time or space, but the concept of fair balance certainly leaves a lot of leeway for interpretation.

For her part, Shaw sees this fair-balance requirement as one favorable aspect of DTC advertising because it means mentioning side effects or other considerations patients might not hear in a physician's office at all.

"I can tell you from experience [that] when a pharmaceutical sales rep pitches to a doctor, we state many benefits and rarely state more than one possible side effect. We make sure that we say whatever is necessary to convince the doctor that we are carrying the best medication out there," she says. While doctors may leave out certain facts when discussing drugs and their side effects with patients, patients can potentially find this information after seeing a drug in a commercial if they do some research and view package inserts online.

"My point is that if DTC helps the patients realize that there are options, there are side effects associated with prescription meds and they need to get informed and ask doctors questions, that is a good thing. But, if a patient sees a commercial on TV and marches into a doctor's office and specifically requests that medication for no other reason than the commercial, they may be receiving a prescription that is not in their best interest," says Shaw, who is now a passionate advocate for informed choices for patients. DTC advertising may be an iteration of the consumer culture we are immersed in, but prescription drugs will never be simply another commodity to brand and market—not when people's lives are at stake.

For Duncan Cross, DTC ads represent a diversion of resources that should be earmarked for patient care. "There is no therapeutic benefit to these ads, and yet every sick person in the country winds up subsidizing them one way or another," he says. To his point, DTC advertising of "blockbuster" drugs, those name-brand top sellers we can all spot the jingles for, has another effect: contributing indirectly and directly to the increasing costs of medical care. In fact, the money spent promoting and marketing big-name drugs is one of the biggest criticisms of DTC advertising. Experts call these lucrative, heavily marketed brand-name drugs "me-too" drugs because they are minor variations of older drugs, ones that are often produced to extend patents on drugs that are about to expire. This way, pharmaceutical companies get exclusive marketing rights for what is essentially the same drug.[29] In a 2004 interview, Dr. Marcia Angell, former editor-in-chief of the *New England Journal of Medicine* and author of *The Truth About the Drug Companies*, explained that me-too drugs don't just cost money in promotions and marketing; they siphon away from the type of true innovation that many patients need.

"If you look at the new drugs marketed over the last six years, 78 percent weren't even new chemical compounds. They were just new combinations or different formulations of old drugs. And 68 percent were classified by the FDA as unlikely to be improvements over drugs already on pharmacy shelves," Dr. Angell said, adding that drug shortages exist in other disease categories because making them is not as profitable as churning out more me-too drugs.

Lack of innovation is especially worrying for patients with rare diseases, who are at an obvious disadvantage since their small populations (two hundred thousand patients or fewer) make them unattractive to drug developers. If all patients are vulnerable in the consumer-Pharma relationship, then patients with rare diseases have the most perilous position. We rely on the Orphan Drug Act, first enacted in 1983, legislation that gives pharmaceutical companies incentives to research and develop medications for rare diseases, which obviously aren't the cash cows that diseases that affect millions more patients are. We risk losing out on true innovation in favor of promotion.

Still, if we hold the idea that culture change happens when people start having conversations, then there is value in this scenario. We are talking about illness more, and potentially embarrassing or stigmatizing chronic health conditions are a regular part of our syntax. What DTC advertising exposes—and social media and patient groups should combat—is that people are not as informed as they need to be if they are getting their information from a thirty-second commercial. When a consumer decides to request a medication based on seeing a TV ad, the self-diagnosis and selection of treatment are placed *before* the clinical and laboratory assessments that would support the diagnosis and choice of treatment. Ideally, the physician would correct the sequence of events, and a comprehensive conversation and appropriate observations and tests would occur based on differential diagnoses.

Since pharmaceutical companies are naturally looking to expand their consumer reach, it is no surprise that they have followed patients and patient organizations into the virtual world. Some do it better (that is, more transparently) than others, and their growing social media presence translates into even more discernment for patients. In an effort to get their products visible, pharmaceutical companies and their PR reps have gone "new school," where the patients are: they are on Twitter, they are on Facebook, they maintain blogs, YouTube channels, and more.

"I believe social networking is a great avenue to explore for health care innovation and product marketing. Since next-generation health and health care is largely about driving behavior change through getting trusted information, where better than Facebook and other similar sites to get the word out virally about new solutions and products and to utilize 'positive peer pressure' for better living? Patients will be able to benefit from higher-value-added products and services and experience real life change," says Tony Chen of FDAzilla, a company that helps professionals work smarter with the FDA by making data usable and actionable.[30] "While old-school companies are still negotiating with their ad firm on a marketing theme for their product launch, new-school companies already have thousands of people using it and giving them feedback for the next version of their product," he says. Some companies have started interacting with patients and thought-leaders in the world of health care social media directly, sponsoring summits and conferences to hear from patients and explore how best to engage with them through social media platforms.

Patient advocacy groups, such an integral part of modern-day patient-hood and culture change when it comes to health care and chronic disease, are caught up in this transparency dynamic, too. When they are legitimate and not biased by funding sources, Barbara Kivowitz calls them "the first oasis for a desperate, thirsty, wandering sick person." Over time, the connections and support patients receive from patient advocacy can help them become advocates themselves and give insight and action back into the system itself.

According to Dr. Adriane Fugh-Berman, an associate professor at Georgetown University and director of Pharmedout, a project at the university's medical center that helps physicians identify and respond to inappropriate drug promotions, there are only about six national consumer advocacy groups that do not take any money from pharmaceutical companies, a conflict of interest that patients shouldn't ignore. It can be difficult to locate sponsorship on some of the sites that do receive funding. Since drug companies have co-opted existing groups without indicating the real sponsor in the past, Fugh-Berman sees as dangerous the potential for this to happen on social networking sites. A 2011 study in the *American Journal of Public Health* found that most advocacy groups that have the appearance of being grassroots organizations fail to disclose the grants they get from pharmaceutical companies. At the same time, these groups have agendas that often overlap with the marketing efforts of their financial supporters. For example, increasing public awareness about a disease or increasing physicians' recognition of it could lead to more sales of treatments and devices designed for that disease.[31] Regulations that require disclosure of gifts to physicians do not extend to patient advocacy groups, something researchers hope will change in the future.

Do the benefits of access to health innovation and communities of patients outweigh the risks of potential conflicts of interest or inappropriate marketing? If patients are aware of any financial relationships between companies and advocacy groups, perhaps yes.

"I'm fine with it, as long as there is transparency," says Rosalind Joffe, the chronic illness life coach from Newton, Massachusetts. Both of her websites, keepworkinggirlfriend.com and cicoach.com, contain ads for services that are relevant to her clients. "In many ways, advertising, blogs, and networking sites are terrific ways for the medical consumer to know what is available," she says. An ad for a product that helps people lift things, which can be a daily struggle with the debilitating effects of multiple sclerosis, is a prime example of the type of ad Joffee would green-light. A patient with multiple sclerosis herself, Joffe was once a spokesperson for Biogen Idec (producer of the multiple sclerosis drug Avonex) at patient education seminars. Avonex was never promoted by any of the speakers, although there were tables that had information about the product.

"Again, I think it's all about transparency," Joffe says. "My website sells my services as a chronic illness coach and the products that help them but it also has lots of free and valuable information . . . folks with chronic illness, in particular, feel susceptible to being 'duped' by false promises or false advertising. I use the Web to promote my services and it's how people have found me and how my business has grown the way it has. There's always a fine line between 'advertising' and 'information.'"

We do indeed live in a culture of consumption, and as patients with chronic illness, we are magnets for health information. We need patient advocacy groups to keep fighting for research and resources, just as we need pharmaceutical companies to strive for drug innovation and authentic dialogue. Collaboration is what makes e-Patient Dave deBronkart's success story possible, what makes participatory medicine a goal for twenty-first-century patients and physicians alike.

"One great challenge we face is the cultural barrier in which some people—providers and patients alike—have built a belief system where clinicians have an almost shamanistic magic to them. In that belief system it's sacrilege or travesty for a patient to have any power. We address this by sharing stories that prove patients truly can bring value to the table, and by refining the point: I helped in my case, but I'm no oncologist, I'm no kidney surgeon, I'm no orthopedic surgeon, I'm no nurse. The point isn't to overthrow doctors; it's that patients can help," says deBronkart. His comments shed perspective on the future of health care in the digital age, but they are also reminiscent of the same type of power balance patients and advocates have sought for decades: not to dismantle the figure of the physician altogether, but to legitimize the patient voice and legitimize the knowledge both parties brings to the relationship.

CHAPTER 9

What Future, at What Cost?

WHEN chef and health columnist Wendell Fowler penned an article lambasting the irresponsibility of an ice cream fundraiser for children with type 1 diabetes in the summer of 2011, he raised the ire of much of the type 1 diabetes community. In assuming the foods they chose were a main cause of their diabetes, Fowler made an entirely too common mistake: he failed to differentiate between type 1 diabetes, an autoimmune disease formerly known as juvenile diabetes, and the much more prevalent type 2 diabetes. Only about 5 percent of patients with diabetes have type 1, which occurs when an autoimmune response attacks the pancreas and it stops producing insulin altogether, meaning patients are insulin-dependent for life.[1] For the millions of Americans who have type 2 diabetes, which is often associated with obesity, they can sometimes manage their condition through changes in diet and lifestyle before they require medication or insulin. The insinuation that type 1 children should not have ice cream or that their lifestyle choices caused their disease angered patients and advocates, who felt that a health columnist and chef should know better than to contribute to the pervasive myth about type 1 diabetes. A viral response played out in social media circles, with type 1 diabetics posting pictures of themselves eating ice cream on Facebook and bloggers indignantly calling Fowler to task for his misinformation.

This incident is just one small example of the uneasiness that surrounds questions of individual responsibility for behavior and illness. Type

1 diabetics don't like being judged for doing something to cause their illness. They don't want to inherit the stereotypes and associations that come with type 2 diabetes, or live with the burden of expectation that if they just ate differently or exercised more, they could "cure" their incurable disease. At the same time, type 2 diabetics don't want to be cast off as lazy or gluttonous and subject to the snap judgments people make about their lifestyle, decisions, and character.

When cookbook author and television chef and personality Paula Deen disclosed she had type 2 diabetes in 2012, news articles, blog posts, and commenters were quick to criticize; after all, Deen's Southern-style cooking is known for its generous amounts of butter, cream, sugar, and other rich, indulgent ingredients. Deen's decision to wait several years to disclose her condition while publicly espousing her high-fat recipes, and her endorsement deal with Novo Nordisk, the pharmaceutical company that manufactures her diabetes medication, added to the maelstrom. Many saw Deen as a hypocrite.

From a public health perspective, there was more at stake than personal feelings about Paula Deen or her motivations for waiting to disclose her condition until her endorsement went public. Leah Roman, whose public health expertise includes a focus on public health and pop culture, considers the situation a lost opportunity for a teachable moment, and such moments, she says, help us "identify a time when our audiences will be more open to prevention, education, and intervention because they see its relevance to their lives. Often the identification and sustainability of teachable moments are supported by media reports on the health and lives of celebrities."[2] What's more, linking Deen's type 2 diabetes exclusively to her diet is what Roman calls a huge simplification of health behavior, which includes environment, socioeconomic status, genetics, and many other factors. "Sometimes that gets left out in the media and in conversation when there is a lot of blaming," Roman says.

"The problem is this: we humans tend to live in shorthand," says Caroline Sheehan. Sheehan is a patient advocate at a federally qualified center that serves low-income patients, and in her personal life she is active in ACT1 Diabetes, a nonprofit diabetes advocacy and support group.

She points to the work of Nobel Prize winners Daniel Kahneman and Amos Tversky and other psychologists who have researched heuristics, which are the frameworks we use to make decisions. "In a sense, they're the only way we can take action and move forward in daily life instead of analyzing every aspect, opinion, and possibility before making a judgment. But in matters of health, heuristics often backfire. It's much easier to assign blame to individuals for their illness, rather than consider the myriad factors that influence it," she says.

When it comes to, say, an obese female patient with type 2 diabetes, too often the immediate assumption is that patient is lazy. But Sheehan points out another framework: What if the woman works two sedentary jobs to support her children and doesn't have any time to exercise or sleep properly? What if her limited food budget means she eats mainly what her kids like to eat, or the fact that her health insurance only covers half her diabetes supplies means she rations her test strips and doesn't test her blood sugar as often as she should? That plot line is a lot more complicated and requires more consideration, even compassion. Yet it isn't the obvious story, the one we are quick to believe or parse out.

"Much too often, I see a parent of a child with type 1 diabetes lashing out against a news story that does not differentiate between type 1 and type 2 in regards to a new treatment or new research, or yet another story on ever-increasing obesity numbers in Western society. It often leads to them perpetuating myths about type 2 diabetes," says Rachel Foster, a diabetes advocate and active blogger who has type 2 diabetes. "For example, 'what my child eats did not contribute to their diagnosis, unlike someone with type 2 diabetes.' This is not necessarily true, as type 2 diabetes is often genetically influenced. The perception that *anyone* eats their way to diabetes should be avoided."

I see her point. I know type 1 diabetics who are overweight and type 2 diabetics who are rail-thin. I know people who developed diabetes as a result of taking steroids to treat other life-threatening diseases, and I know plenty of people who are overweight and don't exercise who breeze through their cardiovascular and glucose tests without a glitch. As a younger patient with type 2 diabetes—she was diagnosed before the age of thirty—Foster lives with many assumptions about her lifestyle, despite that fact that they no longer hold true. Admittedly, she made some poor choices when it came to nutrition and exercise during her twenties, but she acknowledges a strong genetic tendency toward the disease as well. For years now she has maintained a healthy diet and exercises regularly each week, in addition to taking a medication to help manage her disease. To her, the deep divide only serves to distract patients and advocates from the common focal points the two diseases share.

"We forget that both type 1 and type 2 diabetes may lead to the same complications involving the eyes, kidneys, heart, and extremities because the ways in which we came to live with diabetes are different. The focus should be on preventing complications instead of constantly speaking of different names for similar disease processes," she says. "We also use the same blood glucose meters—and in some cases, the same insulin pumps and continuous glucose monitoring devices—and we should all be concerned with the accuracy and safety of such devices." In her words are echoes from across the disease spectrum, from parents of children with autism to patients with autoimmune diseases to cancer advocates. At some point, we need to put aside different definitions, or ideas about causation, and make sure that patients living with diseases right now have access to the medications, devices, and services they need for the best health outcomes.

Is that time now?

Premodern times focused on moralistic attitudes about character and illness, and the twentieth century was the age of the biomedical model and discovery, which makes me wonder how the twenty-first century will play out in terms of chronic illness. With 164 million Americans expected to experience chronic illness by 2025 alone, it will undoubtedly be a century of chronic illness.[3] Perhaps the more pertinent question is, under which theme will we characterize how we *respond* to chronic conditions? Will patients with chronic illness mobilize the way we saw so many groups do in the twentieth century, and will the Internet be their vehicle? Will science yet again tempt us with the answers to the mysteries of illness, as it indicates it might with personalized medicine, genetic testing, and other innovations? If we focus even more on the environment and lifestyle, what are we leaving out?

Using Roy Porter's assertion that disease is no less a social development than the treatments that combat it, we can see quite clearly how changes in the way society works, eats, lives, and moves are connected to our experience of illness.[4] The Industrial Revolution changed the way we lived and worked and, in turn, changed the ways in which we became sick with communicable disease. The shift to a more digital workplace means an increasing gap in socioeconomic status, profound differences in the way we consume goods and services, differences in lifestyle and activity, and differences in quality of and access to health care. If the current state of illness in our country is any indication, prosperity and progress, it seems, come with a cost.[5]

Chronic Disease and Prevention:
Stigma and the Cult of Responsibility

As we saw with the type 1–type 2 diabetes scenario, the distinction between conditions that are largely preventable through changes in behavior and those conditions for which prevention means slowing down disease *progression* is an important one. We can point to diet and exercise regimens as some antidotes for lifestyle-acquired illnesses, but the same approach does not work for, say, the patient with cystic fibrosis (CF), or myriad other autoimmune, rare, or genetic diseases. Certainly there are things these patients can do to improve their health status and minimize long-term complications. The CF patient can stick to daily chest physiotherapy to help clear secretions, can diligently take his or her inhalers, nebulizer treatments, antibiotics, and enzyme supplements to help manage infections and maintain nutrition. These steps will hopefully slow down disease progression, but preventing disease progression is not preventing disease itself.

Advancements in treating and preventing infectious disease and other illnesses contribute to our living long enough to acquire chronic conditions, but the statistics reveal that many of today's pressing health issues—obesity, hypertension, heart disease—are related to the choices we make. Alcohol and smoking, diets high in saturated fats, and lack of physical activity, the "hallmarks of life in the West," have a significant role in the development of ongoing health conditions.[6] Heart disease and type 2 diabetes are not unique to our day and age, but the number of people living with them and the demographics of that patient population have changed. Now, heart disease is the leading cause of death for both men and women in our country,[7] and 23.6 million people live with diabetes (the majority of whom have type 2 diabetes). Another 57 million people teeter on the edge of the disease and are classified as having "pre-diabetes."[8] Almost 60 million Americans are obese, and more than 108 million adults are either obese or overweight, or in other words, about three out of every five Americans carry excess (and unhealthy) weight on their frames.[9]

All the talk about sitting in front of computers, driving instead of walking, and watching television instead of moving around are not just generalizations. Thirty-seven percent of Americans admit they are not physically active, and only three out of ten American adults get the recommended amount of regular physical activity (thirty minutes or more, at least five times a week). Regular, moderate exercise can substantially decrease the risk of developing heart disease, type 2 diabetes, and certain cancers, can help keep cholesterol and blood pressure lower, and can lessen symptoms of anxiety and depression.[10]

By and large, our children are less active than even one previous generation were, too. Children need even more regular physical activity than adults do (sixty minutes a day). For some context, one-quarter of American children watch at least four hours of television per day, and only another 25 percent of American teens reported getting moderate exercise each week.[11] As childhood and teen obesity rises, more children are receiving diagnoses of type 2 diabetes, setting them up for a lifetime of possible complications.[12] More than 10 percent of young children (ages two to five) are classified as overweight, a proportion that has doubled since 1980 (the year I was born), and research shows that from 1999 to 2002, 16 percent of children between ages six and nineteen were overweight, a proportion that has tripled since 1980.[13] By 2008, more than one third of children and adolescents were overweight or obese.[14] A recent analysis in the *Lancet* found that if current trends continue, by the year 2030, nearly half of all Americans will be classified as obese. The population of today's obese children who will grow into adults with weight problems is part of this projection.[15]

With statistics like those, it is clear why health care professionals and public health experts are worried. Consider gout, an inflammatory disease that causes intense pain in toes and other joints. Gout was once called the "disease of kings" because it afflicted the wealthy, who could afford rich indulgent foods and large quantities of alcohol.[16] Now, as more Americans grow older, put on weight, and remain sedentary, gout has become a middle-class affliction. An estimated two to six million Americans now suffer from gout, and the *New York Times* reports that the number of cases is thought to have doubled in the past three decades.[17]

We have come a long way from the repressive cancer personality mentality and the dreaded "C" word so vilified by Susan Sontag, but with our knowledge inevitably comes more responsibility. We know that smoking can cause lung cancer and tanning can cause skin cancer, but the association between lifestyle choices and cancer goes beyond that. Experts believe a full 50 to 75 percent of cancers are associated with lifestyle and behavior; 25 to 30 percent of the major cancers that affect U.S. patients may be the result of poor diet and inactivity.[18] Cancer consists of thousands of diseases, and prevention and risk factors vary among specific diagnoses. This isn't to say that genetics, environment, and other variables aren't at play in the manifestation of cancer. Of course they are, and to assume otherwise is a damaging stance. People with the same basic diet and level of activity can have completely different health outcomes: one may develop diabetes or heart disease or a form of cancer, while the other may encounter only minor health problems. However, educating people about the many types of cancer that have known risk factors is a public health priority.

You can't have a conversation about chronic disease, lifestyle, and responsibility without mentioning the big "P" word: Prevention. In fact, it is one of the most oft-referenced terms in the discourse, from governmental and political writings to public policy. Looking at the big-picture statistics, there is good reason for such focus: each year, seven out of every ten deaths are the result of chronic disease, and five chronic diseases (heart disease, cancer, stroke, diabetes, and chronic obstructive pulmonary disease) with lifestyle associations cause two-thirds of deaths each year. Of the 133 million Americans who live with chronic disease, many have more than just one condition, and collectively, 75 percent of health care spending (an estimated $1 trillion in 2005, for example) is attributable to chronic disease.[19] Unless there is a major system change, the Centers for Medicare and Medicaid estimate that health care spending will double over the course of the next decade, costing us a predicted $4.3 trillion in the year 2017.[20]

The message to change our lifestyle is pervasive, even if the change that follows it is nascent. From First Lady Michelle Obama's "Let's Move!" initiative—one goal of which is to fight childhood obesity—to wellness initiatives and incentives for weight loss sponsored by corporations and by health insurance companies, healthy living and healthy eating are constant cultural conversations. Many health insurance plans now subsidize gym memberships, and coverage of services like nutrition consulting is more common. It is a start, but the scope is much bigger. Preventive measures rest on the assumption that patients have access to adequate and appropriate health care, the resources and knowledge to make changes in diet, opportunities for safe physical activity, and environments that support wellness in all its forms. We aren't helped by the increased portion sizes in restaurants and stores, by the marketing gimmicks and flashy advertising of unhealthy foods, particularly toward children, and by the abundance of processed, nutritionally depleted prepared foods we consume.

In a much different way, our consumer culture has introduced an intellectual shift in regard to nutrition. Best-selling books like Michael Pollan's *The Omnivore's Dilemma* and *In Defense of Food* urge us to abandon processed food substitutes in favor of the real thing—whole, fresh foods— telling us that doing so will benefit our health as well as the environment. Many processed foods have ingredient lists that are several lines long, and a common frame of reference is to point to our grandparents' generation, before relentless marketing campaigns and "food products" replaced freshly cooked meals. The Center for Science in the Public Interest has a comprehensive glossary of food additives it calls "Chemical Cuisine." The list of additives marked in red labeled "Avoid" contains almost two dozen additives, including partially hydrogenated vegetable oil, common in processed foods, and the potentially carcinogenic sodium nitrate and sodium nitrite, which are often used in processed meats—foods that are also often high in saturated fats and sodium.[21]

Pollan's mantra that we should "Eat food. Not too much. Mostly plants," quickly made it from the *New York Times* to food and health bloggers' posts across the Internet.[22] In 2009, *New York Times* food writer Mark Bittman published his "vegan before six P.M." strategy, and the value of a diet lower in animal fats and higher in plant-based proteins was something more than a doctor's suggestion—it was almost trendy.[23] The rise of the "foodie culture" promulgated by shows like *The Next Food Network Star, Iron Chef America, Top Chef,* and many more elevated cooking—and therefore eating—with the general public. It is now fashionable to make stock from scratch, to linger over red wine reductions, and to experiment with fresh vegetables. Farmers' markets are growing in popularity, from bustling urban downtowns to leafy exurbs, and more customers are starting to branch out from local produce and fruits to locally raised, hormone-free meats. These developments are promising, but only as far as their reach extends. If you have the means and awareness to buy locally produced goods at farmers' markets, or the time and resources to make more food from scratch and cut down on processed items, hopefully you will reap the health benefits. If we think back to Caroline Sheehan's example of the overworked, fiscally strapped type 2 diabetic trying to raise a family and keep her disease under control, we begin to see how flimsy the safety net of the "right choices" can be.

Prevention is tied to empowerment—giving people the tools they need to manage their health. Health literacy, an understanding of appropriate technology, access to affordable medications, knowledge and resources to prepare healthful foods, and regular opportunities for exercise are paramount. "We can't goad a person into willingness to take care of themselves; the desire to manage their illness is fundamental and comes from them alone. But beyond that, it becomes a two-pronged effort of individual responsibility and community empowerment through the tools provided," Sheehan says.

Of course, knowledge does not mean action. We might know about calories, nicotine, or the ill health effects of sugary beverages and processed foods, yet we still smoke, or eat too much of the wrong foods. Likewise, we might know the means of transmission of HIV, for example, and what we can do to protect ourselves. AIDS advocate Susan Tannehill said bluntly, "You can *not* get HIV," and yet millions of people continue to get infected. In 2006, the Centers for Disease Control reported 56,300 people were *newly* infected with HIV.[24] Similarly, the patient with multiple sclerosis may know full well that extreme heat or cold exacerbates his or her symptoms but may choose to overdo it in the heat anyway; the patient with celiac disease may know that ingesting even a small amount of gluten could trigger symptoms but may have "just a bite" of bread regardless. And of course implicit in these examples is the assumption that the patient *does* know these things, just like we assume the type 2 diabetic knows enough about the glycemic index to make smart food choices, or the asthmatic understands that environmental pollutants and allergies could be significant triggers for his or her congestion.

Barbara Kivowitz is all too aware of just how precious her socioeconomic status is in terms of her health and her management of chronic pain. She may not be truly wealthy, but as an employed white-collar professional, she has comprehensive health insurance that covers tests considered experimental. She has been able to shop around and consult with specialists at top-tier hospitals in different cities. What's more, her socioeconomic status grants her access to a certain social network, both professionally and personally, and those connections can prove useful when bumping up against a seemingly impermeable health care system.

But what if you don't have such good insurance? What if you can't afford the insurance you do have, or if you lost it and no longer qualify? If you're healthy, maybe you will get lucky and remain that way until your situation changes. But if you have chronic disease and do not have adequate health care, prevention is a luxury that is no longer yours. It's about survival—physically, financially, and emotionally. The greatest economic fear I have is losing my health insurance, and I live in Massachusetts, where a type of universal health insurance already exists. A loss to me is not as black-and-white as having no insurance at all; it could mean less comprehensive health care, and even that nuance could mean several thousand dollars more in bills each year. I am grateful for the excellent health insurance that I work incredibly hard to provide for my family, and even with that, there are always letters to write, explanations to offer, and battles to wage to convince the people in charge of approving claims that preventive care is truly medically necessary. I have an incredible pulmonary specialist, one of the few well versed in my rare lung disease, and access to the most updated diagnostic procedures. That little blue card I carry with me is the difference between life and death, between being productive and being incapacitated, between economic stability and financial catastrophe. My socioeconomic status, propelled largely by education, geography, and similar childhood opportunities, gives me access to the little blue card with the power to determine so much.

As the gap between rich and poor continues to widen, so too does the gap in health and positive health outcomes. The Centers for Disease Control and Prevention defines these health disparities as differences in health outcomes and their determinants between different population segments—typically, along social, environmental, geographic, and demographic lines.[25] Health disparities cover an enormous swath of variables and correlations, much more than what we can discuss here, but some snapshots of the type of disparities that exist should illustrate the breadth of the problem. Air pollution, which can exacerbate asthma, impacts the overall health of people living within its radius. While both rich and poor live and work in areas that have significant levels of air pollution and are affected by it, the fact that racial and ethnic minority groups are more likely than whites to live in urban areas means they continue to experience a larger impact from it. Although heart disease cuts across racial and socioeconomic lines, black men and women are much more likely to die from heart disease than whites; and coronary artery disease and stroke, the leading causes of death in our country, represent the biggest discrepancy in life expectancy among blacks and whites. What's more, rates of preventable hospitalizations increase as income decreases, and black patients are hospitalized for preventable medical issues at more than twice the rate of white patients.[26]

The phrase "poverty is a carcinogen" was coined in 1989 by then director of the National Cancer Institute, Dr. Samuel Broder. More than twenty years later, poverty ranks right up there with smoking and obesity as a cancer-causing agent. In reflecting on the National Cancer Institute's 2011 Facts and Figures report, Dr. J. Leonard Lichtenfeld highlights some of the more startling statistics, starting with the fact that 37 percent of cancer deaths in people between the ages of twenty-seven and sixty-four are associated with poverty. Those living in poverty who also lacked education fared even worse. For example, deaths from lung cancer occur four to five times more often in the least educated patients than they do in the most educated ones. In fact, Dr. Lichtenfeld writes, "Education trumps ethnicity."[27] Individuals with less education tend to have lower incomes. Those with lower incomes face more obstacles to care, including routine preventive health services, and those who lack health insurance are diagnosed with cancer at later stages and therefore face more grim prognoses.[28]

As just a handful of examples illustrate, factors like lack of education, health insurance, and health literacy coupled with numerous environmental contributions and genetics make prevention of disease a loaded topic. There is still another snag in the individual-responsibility-for-behavior thread, though. If we truly are moving away from the biomedical model of disease and are willing to accept that illness, like wellness, does not exist in a vacuum, then we must look at the ramifications of such intense focus on individual choices. Can this emphasis on changing lifestyle and behavior stray into blaming patients for illness and stigmatizing them? Is it just another manifestation of the same pattern repeated throughout history?

Potentially, yes.

"The only downside of making people more aware of individual responsibility is the risk of stigmatizing the overweight and obese. Ironically that stigma is becoming less and less of a risk as the majority of Americans are overweight or obese! The NHLBI [National Heart, Lung, and Blood Institute] recognizes that a five- to ten-percent total body weight loss is sufficient for substantial medical benefits. The idea is not for Americans to hold up anorexic supermodels as our wellness ideal—but rather [to become] strong, fit people at any size (within reason)," says Dr. Val Jones. She raises an interesting point about the lessening of the stigma against the obese. At the other end of the spectrum is the "fat acceptance" movement, which has gained momentum in the twenty-first century thanks to blogs and social media. Advocates for fat acceptance decry the discrimination and stigmatization of people based on their weight and the assignation that weight reflects negative aspects of a person's character.

The prevalence of weight discrimination has increased by 66 percent over the last decade and is now comparable to rates of racial discrimination, especially for women. Widespread beliefs that overweight and obese people are lazy, weak, lack self-discipline, and are less competent mean inequities exist in the workplace, in educational institutions, and in health care facilities.[29] Particularly troubling are attitudes among health care professionals; in one study of primary care physicians, more than 50 percent of them considered their obese patients to be unattractive and noncompliant, while one third described them as sloppy and weak-willed. Physicians revealed that they considered their patients' weight problems to be primarily a behavioral issue, brought on by overeating and inadequate exercise.[30] Individuals pick up on these attitudes, whether in health care settings or workplace environments, and out of a possible twenty sources of stigma, patients in one study ranked physicians as the second most common source. Emotional distance between patient and physician is a recurrent theme in the social history of chronic illness, and in this case, it is not too difficult to imagine that the obese patient who picks up on his or her physician's judgment or disdain may not be too forthcoming. As soon as conversations about health (physical *and* psychosocial) break down, the likelihood of a positive health outcome does, too.

It seems to be human nature to want to scapegoat people who have AIDS or lung cancer and other highly stigmatized diseases as being at fault for engaging in risky behavior. We tend to be uncomfortable with the knowledge that some people who get lung cancer never smoked, for example, because that means it isn't something that only happens to other people—other people making choices *we* wouldn't. Intellectually, of course, we know we aren't immune from illness. As many patients with chronic illness have pointed out in this book, we don't like to acknowledge some health problems that won't go away, that stretch beyond the limits of even the most advanced medical resources and can't be cured.

When I was a college student at Georgetown University, the humid, swampy weather of Washington, D.C., made my daily struggle to breathe even more challenging. Sometimes it felt like I was inhaling sludge, and no matter what I did, I couldn't get more than shallow breaths. I was hospitalized much more frequently during my three years in D.C. than I was the year I studied abroad in Dublin, Ireland, where the weather was more consistent (even if rainy) and the air was much less humid. The physical environment impacts my symptoms in a very real way. However, as researchers and patients interested in parsing out the causes of disease can attest, the term "environment" has a much broader meaning than what we typically associate with the word. When it comes to matters of health and wellness, it includes where we dwell (urban, suburban, exurban, or rural setting), what degree and type of air pollution we're exposed to, what types of plastics we use to store and cook food, what sweeteners we put in our coffee, and more.

Asthma is a revealing disease to explore in this context. Twenty million Americans—one out of every five—have asthma, and it is the most common chronic disease in childhood; nearly five million asthma patients are under the age of eighteen.[31] It is expensive, both in terms of emergency room visits and hospitalizations and in terms of lost wages and productivity. Forty thousand Americans stay out of work or school each day due to asthma symptoms, and every day, five thousand patients visit emergency rooms because of it and one thousand people are admitted to hospitals.[32] Asthma has a strong genetic component, but its symptoms and severity are greatly influenced by environment. Dust, mold, smog, chemicals, fragrances, exhaust, and other environmental triggers can cause or exacerbate asthma attacks; a 2010 study in the *Journal of Allergy and Clinical Immunology* found that air pollution was linked to suppressed immune function that worsened the severity of asthma attacks in children.[33]

There is some compelling research that suggests that for many with chronic illnesses, particularly autoimmune diseases, the chemicals that are such an omnipresent part of our world play a role, too. In *The Autoimmune Epidemic*, Donna Jackson Nakazawa takes readers on an intense journey to uncover how what we breathe, what we consume, and what we absorb can make our immune systems go haywire. To augment her point, Nakazawa highlights statistics like these: In 2005, the Centers for Disease Control and Prevention found a staggering 287 pollutants and industrial chemicals in the fetal cord blood from ten newborns around the country.[34] A 2007 study examining the association between exposure to chemicals in the workplace and developing certain systemic autoimmune disease found that farmers who worked with crops and were exposed to pesticides were more likely to die from autoimmune disease,[35] and a 2006 study using hospital data found that patients with rheumatoid arthritis or lupus who breathe in air polluted with heavy particles for a year or longer face a 22 percent increase in the risk of dying from their disease.[36] Though merely a sampling of the exhaustive research she supplies, these facts are persuasive evidence that the chemicals that have become ubiquitous in our environment also become part of our physiology. If the way we live is implicated in heart disease or type 2 diabetes, it is no less implicated in the misfirings and disruptions of the immune system that can result in autoimmune diseases.

"The ever-increasing severity and number of illnesses probably doesn't speak too well for our society. If we didn't feel such pressure to ignore symptoms or lead such high-stress lives, maybe more cases of serious illness would be nipped in the bud; maybe less would develop in the first place. If we put more focus on leading balanced lives—if we valued rest, relaxation, nutrition, and exercise in the same way that we seem to value stress—we would undoubtedly be a healthier society as a whole," observes Jennifer Crystal, whose neurological Lyme disease has forced her to build more balance into her personal life.

Not surprisingly, stress and autoimmune diseases are linked as well. While even healthy people can attest to the toll stressful life events can take on physical health, when it comes to chronic illness and in particular autoimmune disease, the relationship between stress and disease is notable.

Stress alone is not what causes illness, an association many patients chafe under in their doctors' offices, but rather that stress often worsens the symptoms and the progression of a disease. Stress did not cause the genetic mutation that means the cilia I need in my lungs do not work, nor does it cause the mucus that chokes me, or the infections I pick up so easily from those around me. However, when I am unusually stressed, worried, or overworked and I don't sleep well and I push myself beyond my limits, my infections last longer, my oxygen saturation isn't as good, and my energy is strained. For patients with multiple sclerosis and rheumatoid arthritis, stress is linked with an increased risk of flares and the onset and worsening of symptoms, respectively.[37]

Does this mean we can simply chalk some diseases up to a polluted world, or to systemic stress overload? No. To do so would be to overlook the genetic predisposition, randomness, and confluence of all of these factors that have been responsible for these diseases throughout the ages. However, given the drastic changes in lifestyle, manufacturing, and behavior in the past sixty years or so, we cannot look at increased rates of illness without this data in mind.

The other component in the chronic illness equation is, of course, genetics. As a patient with a genetic lung disease, I am all too familiar with the vagaries of inherited illness. No one else in my family has PCD, although my uncle and I share a diagnosis of celiac disease, which does have a genetic component to it. Some patients have a genetic predisposition toward a disease (such as type 2 diabetes or heart disease) that tips them over into the disease category, even if their lifestyle and environmental factors themselves might not have. But close to 20 percent of people living with chronic disease have diseases that are *not* attributed to lifestyle. For them, the genetic component of illness, not prevention and not environment, is of utmost importance. More than that, this genetic component is a source of stigma itself. I've had strangers, health care professionals, and even family members question whether I should have a child because of my genetic background. In the blogosphere, I know of patients with type 1 diabetes and patients with other diseases that have a genetic component— even if their case isn't directly inherited—who have been told similar

things: we don't have the right to pass on our "faulty" genes. Such comments leave me indignant, but they do not surprise me, not anymore. I could
craft lengthy rebuttals about ignorance, or spout facts about inheritability
versus the many conditions we acquire through our lifetimes, or point to
the achievements people with illness have met. Parenting, working, writing, participating in my community, and managing those very conditions
that bring judgment so I can do each of these things are a better use of
my time.

When the human genome was fully mapped in 2003, its potential to
unravel the mysteries of so many diseases was exhilarating. Now, personalized medicine uses genetic information to develop more targeted drugs.
You can send your saliva off in a specially designed kit to get a DNA analysis done of your risk for acquiring diseases. With this information you can
seek out others just like you, you can research conditions more fully to assess your risk, and in the case of lethal diseases like Huntington's, you can
find out whether or not you possess the gene that will someday manifest
this brutal disease. Understanding why diseases happen is a critical step in
targeting better treatment for them, perhaps even in allowing for curative
measures someday.

It is in matters of DNA research that informed consent is again a controversial topic. Science writer Amy Harmon, who authored a Pulitzer
Prize–winning series on the impact of genetic technology for the *New
York Times*, reports that today's scientists struggle with how to apply the
concept of informed consent to genetic research. Federal courts have ruled
that once cells leave the body, we don't have property rights to them, but
courts do uphold our right to know how those cells will be used. Cases in
which study participants find out their DNA is being used for purposes
beyond what they were told raise important questions for the future. Can
we ensure DNA remains anonymous? What is the best way to get voluntary consent? What happens if scientists use DNA to study diseases or
conditions the individuals don't want to know more about?[38] Science moves
us one step closer to eliminating the stigma of illness by giving us more
information, but technology opens up new opportunities for our health to
be a source of discrimination.

Similarly, stem cell research also has the potential to yield huge leaps in understanding and treating chronic and debilitating diseases. It is highly politicized in nature; President Barack Obama overturned George W. Bush's federal funding ban within months of taking office in 2009, to the exultation of many scientists and patients, and the issue quickly became entrenched in red state–blue state politics. Stem cells are undifferentiated, which means that under the right conditions, they can grow into specific types of cells—heart, lung, tissue, etc.—and can replace unhealthy, dying cells. When applied to diseases like cancer, heart disease, and diabetes, as well as to patients with spinal cord injuries and other conditions, such re-generation could radically alter treatments and outcomes.[39] Since many stem cells are harvested from embryos used in in-vitro fertilization, stem cell research is a hotly contested issue. In previous decades, we had Karen Ann Quinlan and the right to die, and Terry Schiavo and the right to life; and for some, stem cell research is wrapped up in the same conversation about abortion, right to life, and the government's role in shaping science policy. In what some researchers fear as a sign of the return to Bush's "Dark Ages," in 2011, nearly all Republican presidential candidates said they were in favor of limiting President Obama's broadened funding of embry-onic stem cell research.[40] For patients and families waiting for a break-through, the issue is as intensely personal as it is political for others.

Barbara Kivowitz believes the degree to which we view illness as a value itself reflects directly back to our broader cultural priorities. If illness and death are seen as natural processes of living, then we look at patients differently than if illness is seen primarily as a weakness or failing. Stigma and blame have been ascribed to individuals for centuries, whether we're looking at the slum-dweller who became the prevailing image of the tuber-culosis patient in the nineteenth century, the upper-middle-class female patient with fibromyalgia who stands as a symbol of psychosomatic anxiety, or the patient with HIV or Hepatitis C whose infections are the conse-quences of risky behavior. In the twenty-first century, as emphasis on life-style's role in illness increases, the scope of patients who live with diseases are increasingly held responsible for managing their illness through behav-ior choices. The physical, emotional, and economic toll of chronic disease means prevention will be a constant theme. Yet as we've seen, the factors that go into the prevention and progression of many diseases—health disparities, socioeconomic status, access to health care, environment, and genetics, to name some—make it much more complicated than snap judgments would have it seem. I am especially drawn to the perspective that as humans, we tend to live in the shorthand. The long view is much more difficult, but it is what is required of us if we are to move away from these deeply entrenched views on illness, character, and suffering.

Patient Advocacy and Health Care Reform

The social history of modern chronic illness is also inevitably a history of activism. Breakthroughs like the triple-drug cocktail for HIV, workplace accommodations for those disabled by their chronic illnesses, informed consent for clinical trials, and disclosure of diagnosis were due in large part to patient advocacy. Over the last several decades, we've seen groups set aside specific agendas and mobilize for universal gains. One of the biggest issues affecting people with chronic illness right now is health insurance. So where were the protests, the mobilization, and the impassioned action during the tenuous battle for health care reform in 2010? If health insurance and access to care isn't a rallying point for patients with chronic illness, what is?

The Patient Protection and Affordable Care Act, the end result of the bipartisan squabble over health care reform, has been criticized by some as not doing enough for people with chronic illness and by many others as being a bloated attempt at reform that will end up bankrupting the system further. The Supreme Court upheld its constitutionality in 2012, though the debate is far from over. There are reasons many presidents have tried to reform health care in this country for decades and have not been successful. Powerful insurance lobbies, deeply entrenched political positions on the size and scope of government, and a whole host of conflicting agendas and priorities on state and federal levels are just some of the challenges. No one disputes that health care is too expensive and too inefficient in this country, nor that if patients have adequate insurance and can access preventive care, both health outcomes and health care spending will improve. What we can't seem to agree on—and even after President Obama signed the Act into law, what we *still* don't agree on—is the best way to make this happen. While some remain steadfast that a true single-payer system like we see in Canada or the United Kingdom is the only way to offer equal, adequate care, on the other end of the spectrum, critics want health insurance to remain a private enterprise.

Much is at stake for patients with chronic illness in the Patient Protection and Affordable Care Act, including an end to lifetime caps on coverage by insurers, a huge issue for patients with ongoing and expensive chronic conditions. Companies can no longer deny coverage based on pre-existing conditions, which is perhaps the most important change for people with chronic illness, since chronic illness is the embodiment of a preexisting condition. It also ensures that insurance companies offer coverage to children with preexisting illness. It extends coverage to young adults on their parents' plans through the age of twenty-six, including young adults who are married or students. Insurance exchanges set up for individuals and small businesses will allow them to look for competitively priced plans they can afford. Health insurance is now compulsory, and those who don't purchase it will face graduated tax penalties.[41]

It is the mandate that individuals must purchase health insurance that concerns opponents, as well as the tax penalties and worries that governmental oversight will not be up to the task of managing such an enormous, intricate system. ("Look at Medicare!" they claim, or at the beleaguered Social Security system; if the government can't handle that, how can it handle health care for all?) For patients with chronic illness who longed for a true universal system—the single-payer route—the Affordable Care Act is a step, but it is not the guarantee they'd hoped it would be.

E-Patient Dave reminds us that cultural change, however slow to evolve, begins with the conversations people have about what is possible. In that light, I see something not just salvageable but redeemable from our imperfect solution.

Today's debate takes place within a long-standing context of advocacy for health care reform. In the early twentieth century, health insurance and employment were closely linked. Progressive reformers wanted to protect workers, who lost too much of their wage and too often sank into poverty due to sickness. In fact, Theodore Roosevelt's "insurgent Progressive party" called for compulsory health insurance as far back as 1912.[42] Suffragists also took on the cause, since health insurance included maternity benefits for female laborers, but any momentum was squashed by a powerful conflagration of elites: physicians, business leaders, insurance companies, and conservative politicians.[43] (An eerily familiar pattern, no?) Depression-era politics and the New Deal ushered in a period of upheaval, when social movements to protect workers and provide economic security increased. Given the steep toll exacted by the Great Depression, economic recovery was prioritized over medical care.[44] Nowadays, the response to a similar argument about our current economic state is that appropriate medical care is an essential part of recovery.

Momentum picked up in the 1940s, when the cost of medical care became burdensome enough for labor unions to enter the fight. Labor backed proposed legislation to create a national medical insurance program that would be financed through Social Security payroll taxes, a bill that enjoyed President Harry Truman's support. However, as author Beatrix Hoffman points out, the opportunity to mobilize from the grassroots was lost when labor leaders and politicians felt they did not need the support or inclusion of labor union member themselves.[45] Top-down mobilization is rarely successful in meeting the needs of the people it is meant to represent.

Another window of opportunity emerged in the 1960s during the battle over Medicare. Civil rights activists saw the protections Medicare offered elderly Americans as part of a larger war on poverty, and labor unions endorsed the legislation. Elderly people made more sympathetic victims than other groups, and made it much harder for influential groups like the American Medical Association to discredit them. Now, the image of reform wasn't the face of a progressive suffragette, a labor boss, or a wily politician—it was someone's grandmother or grandfather. The elderly would come to represent a strong and well-populated arm of support for health care reform.[46] Yet again the relationship between economics and health care became evident in the 1980s and '90s, when the rising cost of the uninsured made reform a popular, accepted concept once more. Hoffman attributes the failure of the Clinton presidency to enact health care reform to its reliance on elite decision making that left out the grassroots members, only consulting citizens when the plan had already been drafted.[47]

With all this in mind, let's consider the situation in 2010: steep economic decline and unemployment. Staggering national debt and soaring health care costs, especially for those with chronic illness. Dissatisfaction and outrage over lapses in coverage, denial of claims, and other health insurance woes. With nearly half the country living with chronic illness, this should have been a catalyst moment for patients with chronic illness.

"If 75 percent of health care spending goes to the chronically ill, then health care reform is fundamentally about sick people. Yet the organizations that ostensibly advocate for and empower us did nothing. It still makes me angry. One of the organizations I used to belong to even prohibited its members from discussing 'political' issues in their discussion board. A few of us fought against that online, but meanwhile the organization itself was absolutely silent; not even a link or notice on its home page that the debate was going on," says Duncan Cross.

So where were all the protesters and demonstrations, why weren't people lying in the streets like they did during the disability rights movement in the 1970s? Dr. Joe Wright asked me this question one summer evening in 2009, during the windup to health care reform. I thought about this as I watched the drama over health care reform unfold, and as I watched President Obama sign the bill into law from my hospital bed, where I was twelve weeks pregnant and fighting to breathe and keep my baby safe. (Tweeting it, of course, as much as my poorly placed IV allowed me to type). I've thought about it as I researched and wrote about past reform movements, and various successes and challenges they've met.

If we didn't mobilize in a significant way for health care reform, an issue that had such clear relevance, will chronic illness as a whole ever see the same type of mobilization we saw with other patient and activist populations? Among the many patients, physicians, and experts I spoke with in writing this book over the course of several years, the resounding consensus is no. There are so many different diseases under the umbrella term "chronic illness," and we don't often want to align ourselves with other patients, especially those who may have acquired their disease differently. Research and funding is hard-won, especially in this economic climate, and it is easy to see why sharing a piece of the research checkbook is unappealing. We need different trials, different breakthroughs, and different methods to meet the requirements of our disparate diseases. Highlighting one of the biggest stumbling blocks for advocacy groups, Wright points out that if you are arguing not only over the treatment of disease but also over its cause, you are fighting on several fronts at once. Focusing on a singular purpose was a definitive marker of success for prominent HIV/ AIDS groups, as it was for breast cancer activism and other specialty groups. When the goals become fragmented and people need to defend, justify, or explore the cause of disease as well as champion for various rights, something has to give.

I wonder too about Kairol Rosenthal's concerns about what she calls "slacktivism." Certainly, I read impassioned blog posts about health care reform and followed exuberant Twitter feeds and Facebook messages when the legislation passed. I *know* people with chronic illness were excited, even transformed, by this development. There were a lot of groups and associations who publicly supported the reform, and who tirelessly made their case on economic, health, and moral grounds. If you weren't on social media, if you didn't read the statistics and the arguments, and if you didn't feel connected to people who were as outraged as you were over the state of health insurance in this country, where would you find the momentum? Or, if you were someone who was active on these channels, did it seem enough to "like" the posts or re-Tweet the analysis? Have we lost a sense of urgency due to the immediacy of our message? When I think about the protests and upheaval of the Arab Spring, many of which leapt from smart-phone screens and laptops into crowded public squares, I am reminded that virtual activism is a complement to, not a replacement for, the nuts-and-bolts activism that has yielded so many successes for specific populations of patients.

One sultry summer evening in 2008 stands out in my memory. My husband and I had traveled from Boston to Washington, D.C., to attend the wedding of one of my college friends. It was my first extended trip back to D.C. since I'd graduated, and in the time between, I'd seen the inside of yet another ICU, I'd finally been given correct diagnoses for several of my diseases, and I'd started daily chest physiotherapy and other treatments that drastically improved my quality of life. I'd attended graduate school, fallen in love, then landed an agent and a book deal. My life was full, and with more accurate information on my conditions and how to slow down their progression, I had every reason to believe I would continue to be a fulfilled, productive professional.

I remember donning the heels I so infrequently wear, and a turquoise cocktail dress purchased for this event. I was excited for a great evening watching our friends get married and connecting with college acquaintances I hadn't seen in years. I'd finished the complete draft of my first book on chronic illness and young adults that very morning, holing up in our hotel room while my husband checked out the National Mall. I was exhilarated, I was dressed up, I was in a good place. *I passed*, as far as I was concerned. From all outward appearances, and in my own head and heart in the moment, I was an inveterate member of the kingdom of the well.

As we sipped wine and lingered over the fruit and cheeses during the cocktail hour, we struck up a casual conversation with another young couple. They were impeccably dressed and had impressive professional pedigrees. I don't remember how the topic came up, because I know I didn't volunteer any information, nor did I share any of my own details, but somehow, chronic illness was mentioned.

Out of nowhere, the well-heeled young man with the prestigious degree and the crisp suit and the winning smile said something incredibly ugly—something along the lines of, he'd *never* marry someone with a chronic illness. Why would anyone?

Stupefied, we stared at him and stammered some sort of pat response. My cheeks and neck were burning (they are my tell), and my normally re-served husband looked like he was struggling not to burst. We didn't want to make a scene; we didn't want to delve into something so personal and so vulnerable with strangers who were outrageously confident in their cal-lousness. I looked at his fiancée, with her lithe, willowy frame, her toned, capable arms, her tanned, glowing skin. I thought about all I knew—how millions of women didn't manifest autoimmune and chronic diseases until their twenties and thirties; how chronic illness can sneak up on otherwise healthy people without notice; how many marriages crumble in the face of the overwhelming demands of chronic illness. *Good luck*, I thought to my-self. At the time, my silent words were lobbed toward the young woman with the dark hair and the lilac dress, the woman engaged to a man who didn't seem to believe that people with illnesses were worth sticking around for, or investing in. May she be lucky enough to avoid what millions of other women haven't, and won't.

Years later, I realize I really should have directed my internal mono-logue at both of them. "Chronic illness" is a phrase with no end of mean-ings, one definition stretched over thousands of diseases. It will seep into nearly all of our lives at some point.

Before we dove into Plato and the plagues, before anesthesia and antibiot-ics, before vaccines, organ transplants, and informed consent, before we explored advocacy movements and "new" diseases, and before we saw how technology changed the way we approach the medical establishment, we met two patients: Melissa McLaughlin and Emerson Miller. A few years ago, I considered both their narratives archetypal snapshots of current-day chronic disease. First there was the female patient living with pain whose suffering is somehow less valid because her diagnoses are not as concrete, and because as a young woman, she is seen to be a less reliable narrator of her circumstances. Next, there was the infectious-disease patient whose suffering was also disparaged, but for different prejudices. The two snap-shots represented inscrutable illness versus individual responsibility for be-havior, two of the most pervasive themes in present-day disease, right next to each other.

And they *are* archetypal snapshots, they are successful foils. But what I realize now is that their stories are much more than representations of present-day illness. Our understanding of disease and how it spreads has certainly evolved, but the stereotypes, assumptions, and challenges their narratives pose could apply to the experience of illness across the ages and across the disease spectrum. Have we failed to evolve when it comes to perceptions of illness? Are we that predictable in our fears and insecu-rities, or are we simply adapting to subtle patterns in the only way we know how?

While the fundamental definition of chronic illness hasn't changed, the scope of what is considered chronic has, and what, if anything, does that mean for the patient living with chronic illness? We've seen numerous reasons for the widening scope: We're living longer because we're not dying from communicable disease. We have better technology so we can detect and treat certain conditions earlier and more effectively, and can connect with one another and access information with greater ease. We live in an increasingly consumerist culture where both drugs and the conditions they treat are marketable commodities. We suffer from a dizzying number of preventable diseases at least in part because of unhealthy lifestyles. We are surrounded by chemicals and pollution, and live with economic, pro-fessional, personal, and political stress.

Susan Sontag's powerful image of the division between the kingdom of the well and the kingdom of the sick spoke to me so deeply precisely because of this widening scope. Ultimately, if more and more people dwell in this "night-side of life," do the specific reasons for how we got here mat-ter? I am not convinced they do.

Since I first began writing about chronic illness almost a decade ago, I've clung to the universals, and to the idea that the individual patient's experience with chronic illness is in many ways a universal one. We want to feel better, even if that does not include a cure. We want to feel respected by the fast-paced society we live in, and we want to feel respected by the health care professionals whose job it is to provide the best health outcome possible. We may feel far removed from the patients of medicine's and literature's past, but we're confronted with many of the same frustrations and desires. We want science to give us clues when we're surrounded by darkness, but we do not want to be reduced to impersonal statistics. There are many pieces to our health narratives: the subjective experience of living with illness; clinical observations; environment, lifestyle, and access to health care and health information; political agendas and conflicts of interest in research and funding. More than ever, the onus is on the patient to take part in his or her narrative, to mesh the science that diagnoses and treats us with the culture and technology that has the potential to heal us.

Perhaps that's really the distinction that matters: even if we never find cures for what ails us, can we experience healing? If centuries of illness and advancement tell us anything, then the combination of knowledge, collaboration, and empowerment are a start.

Acknowledgments

I'D like to acknowledge my agent, Matthew Carnicelli, for his enthusiasm for this book and for his intellectual and emotional engagement in it. Jackie Johnson, George Gibson, and the great team at Walker Books gave me the time to dig into questions that I didn't know the answers to but really wanted to find out, and the space to try and make sense of what I discovered. Really, can any nonfiction writer ask for more than that?

This writing process has involved a lot of discussion, research, and reading. Over the course of several years, I've been fortunate to have many patients and health care professionals give me their time and insights. This book is unquestionably richer and more complex thanks to these conversations, and I would like to especially acknowledge Cynthia Toussaint, Dr. Sarah Whitman, Melissa McLaughlin, Barbara Kivowitz, Alicia Cornwell, Janet Geddis, Emerson Miller, Dr. Joe Wright, Amy Brightfield, Jennifer Shaw, Dr. Kevin Pho, Dr. Val Jones, Dr. Gwenn O'Keefe, Susan Tannehill, Phyllis Greenberger, Ginger Taylor, Gina Terrasi Gallagher, Duncan Cross, Dr. Barry Popkin, Rosalind Joffe, Tony Chen, Dr. Adriane Fugh-Berman, Caroline Sheehan, Rachel Foster, e-Patient Dave deBronkart, Jennifer Crystal, Britta Bloomquist, Kairol Rosenthal, Leah Roman, Karen Weintraub, Aviva Brandt, and others.

I'd like to thank the intrepid Rebecca Viola for her all her efforts. She is a skilled researcher and a thoughtful reader. Alice Sapienza and Christen

Enos also tackled different versions of this manuscript and offered truly helpful feedback.

Numerous books and articles are cited in these pages, but I want to take a moment to acknowledge the writers whose expertise truly informed this manuscript. Susan Sontag's *Illness as Metaphor* was the initial spark that set this inquiry in motion years ago: How does language influence the illness experience, and what does the widening scope of chronic illness, despite its somewhat static definition, mean for patients? I am also indebted to the works of Roy Porter, David B. Morris, David J. Rothman, Paula Kamen, and Carl Elliott, among others.

Lastly, I'd like to thank my family and close friends for their contribution to this effort and for their understanding of the idiosyncrasies of a writer's life. My husband, John, did a lot of reading and even more listening, and my daughter, whose birth and babyhood coincided with the writing of this book, was both a constant source of inspiration and motivation and a most cooperative companion.

Notes

INTRODUCTION

1. "About the Crisis," Partnership to Fight Chronic Disease, www.fightchronicdis
   ease.org/issues/about.cfm.
2. "SWHR Timeline," Society for Women's Health Research, www.womenshealth
   research.org/site/PageServer?pagename=about_timeline.
3. Porter, *The Greatest Benefit to Mankind*, 15.
4. Sontag, *Illness as Metaphor and AIDS and Its Metaphors*, 3.
5. Porter, *Greatest Benefit to Mankind*, 29.

CHAPTER 1: FROM PLATO TO POLIO

1. Wall, *Encounters with the Invisible*, 8.
2. Kamen, *All in My Head*, 90.
3. Sontag, *Illness as Metaphor*, 6.
4. Partnership to Fight Chronic Disease, "The Growing Crisis of Chronic
   Disease."
5. Kamen, *All in My Head*, 63.
6. Morris, "How To Speak Postmodern," 1.
7. Ibid., 2.
8. Ibid.
9. Adler, *Medical Firsts*, 8.
10. Ibid., 9.
11. Ibid., 10–11.
12. Ibid., 11.
13. Porter, *Greatest Benefit to Mankind*, 56.
14. Bergdolt, *Wellbeing*, 37–38.
15. Ibid., 38.

16. Ibid., 39.
17. Kennedy, *A Brief History of Disease*, 28.
18. Ibid.
19. Porter, *Greatest Benefit to Mankind*, 84.
20. Ibid.
21. Kennedy, *A Brief History of Disease*, 33.
22. Herek, "Thinking About AIDS and Stigma," 595.
23. Kennedy, *A Brief History of Disease*, 76.
24. Porter, *Greatest Benefit to Mankind*, 122–123.
25. Ibid., 123.
26. Ibid., 125.
27. Ibid., 130.
28. Ibid., 257.
29. Kelly, *Medicine Becomes a Science*, 1.
30. Ibid.
31. Ibid., 8.
32. Porter, *Blood and Guts*, 44.
33. Kelly, *Medicine Becomes a Science*, 12.
34. Sontag, *Illness as Metaphor*, 14–15.
35. Maugham, "Sanatorium," 545.
36. Kelly, *Medicine Becomes a Science*, 24–25.
37. United States Department of Health and Human Services, "The Great Pandemic," http://1918.pandemicflu.gov/the_pandemic/04.htm.
38. Grob, *The Deadly Truth*, 264.
39. Porter, *Greatest Benefit to Mankind*, 15.
40. Ibid.
41. Kelly, *Medicine Becomes a Science*, 84.
42. Ibid.
43. Grob, *The Deadly Truth*, 192.
44. Kelly, *Medicine Becomes a Science*, 85.
45. Porter, *Greatest Benefit to Mankind*, 277.
46. Grob, *The Deadly Truth*, 245.

CHAPTER 2: AN AWAKENING

1. Roberts, "The Commission on Chronic Illness," 296.
2. Ibid., 295.
3. Ibid., 296.
4. Ibid.
5. Sidell, "Adult Adjustment to Chronic Illness," 6.
6. Joffe, "Is This Duo Doable?"
7. Sidell, "Adult Adjustment to Chronic Illness," 2.

8. Elliott, *Better than Well*, 44.

9. Nakazawa, *The Autoimmune Epidemic*, 24.

10. Ibid., 36.

11. Ibid., 38.

12. Centers for Disease Control and Prevention, "Chronic Disease Overview," www.cdc.gov/chronicdisease/overview/index.htm.

13. Ibid.

14. Rao, "Looking Back and Looking Forward," *Preventing Chronic Disease.*

15. Rothman, *Strangers at the Bedside*, 51–53.

16. Sontag, *Illness as Metaphor*, 64–65.

17. National Institutes of Health, "The 1971 National Cancer Act: Investment in the Future," www.nih.gov/news/pr/mar97/nci-26c.htm.

18. Rothman, *Strangers at the Bedside*, 1.

19. Ibid., 16.

20. Ibid., 30.

21. Ibid., 15.

22. Ibid.

23. Ibid., 144.

24. NPR, "Remembering the Tuskegee Experiment," www.npr.org/programs/morning/features/2002/jul/tuskegee/.

25. Centers for Disease Control and Prevention, "The Tusekegee Timeline," www.cdc.gov/tuskegee/timeline.htm.

26. NPR, "Remembering the Tuskegee Experiment."

27. Skloot, *The Immortal Life of Henrietta Lacks*, 4.

28. Rothman, *Strangers at the Bedside*, 3.

29. National Institutes of Health, "Timeline of Laws," http://history.nih.gov/about/timelines_laws_human.html#1949.

30. Rothman, *Strangers at the Bedside*, 155.

31. Lepore, "The Politics of Death," 64.

32. National Hospice and Palliative Care Organization, "NHPCO Facts and Figures," 5.

33. Long, "June 11, 1985: Karen Ann Quinlan Dies," www.wired.com/science/discoveries/news/2008/06/dayintech_0611.

34. Lepore, "The Politics of Death," 66.

35. Centers for Medicare and Medicaid Services, "Tracing the History of CMS Programs," 1.

36. Ibid., 3–4.

37. Daaleman, "Reorganizing Medicare."

38. Centers for Medicare and Medicaid Services, "Tracing the History of CMS Programs," 5.

39. Rothman, *Strangers at the Bedside*, 11.

CHAPTER 3: DISABILITY RIGHTS, CIVIL RIGHTS,
AND CHRONIC ILLNESS

1. Wendell, "Unhealthy Disabled," 19.
2. Ibid., 21.
3. Ibid., 25.
4. Goffman, *Stigma: Notes On the Management of Spoiled Identity*, 4.
5. Disability Rights and Independent Living Movement, "Introduction," http://bancroft.berkeley.edu/collections/drilm/introduction.html.
6. King, *Pink Ribbons, Inc.*, 106.
7. Quigley, "Hospitals and the Civil Rights Act of 1964," 455.
8. Ibid., 457.
9. Hoffman, "Health Care Reform and Social Movements," 80.
10. Disability Rights and Independent Living Movement, "Timeline," http://bancroft.berkeley.edu/collections/drilm/resources/timeline.html.
11. Barnartt and Scotch, *Disability Protests*, 18.
12. Rothman, *Stranger at the Bedside*, 205.
13. Disability Rights and Independent Living Movement, "Timeline."
14. Minnesota Statewide Independent Living Council, "A Chronology of the Disability Rights Movements," www.mnsilc.org/chronology.htm.
15. NPR, "A Look Back At 'Section 504,'" www.npr.org/programs/wesun/features/2002/504/.
16. Disability Rights and Independent Living Movement, "Timeline."
17. Ibid.
18. Wendell, "Unhealthy Disabled," 31.
19. Ibid.
20. Disability Rights and Independent Living Movement, "Timeline."

CHAPTER 4: THE WOMEN'S HEALTH MOVEMENT AND
PATIENT EMPOWERMENT

1. Kamen, *All in My Head*, 98.
2. Gilman, "The Yellow Wallpaper," www.library.csi.cuny.edu/dept/history/lavender/wallpaper.html.
3. U.S. Department of Health and Human Services, "A Century of Women's Health," 17.
4. Kaysen, *The Camera My Mother Gave Me*, 63.
5. Ibid.
6. Barnartt and Scotch, *Disability Protests*, 20.
7. Womenshealth.gov, "Infertility: Frequently Asked Questions," www.womenshealth.gov/faq/infertility.cfm#b.
8. American Autoimmune Related Diseases Association, "Autoimmunity: A Major Women's Health Issue," www.aarda.org/women_and_autoimmunity.php.

9. Ibid.

10. U.S. Department of Health and Human Services, "A Century of Women's Health," 9.

11. Hoffman, "Health Care Reform and Social Movements," 75.

12. King, *Pink Ribbons, Inc.*, xiii.

13. Morgen, *Into Our Own Hands*, x.

14. National Organization for Women, "NOW FAQs," www.now.org/organization /faq.html#found.

15. U.S. Department of Health and Human Services, "A Century of Women's Health," 3.

16. Ibid., 19.

17. Morgen, *Into Our Own Hands*, 4.

18. Morgen, *Into Our Own Hands*, 4–5.

19. Ruzek, "Transforming Doctor-Patient Relationships," 182.

20. Ibid.

21. Rothman, *Strangers at the Bedside*, 144.

22. Ibid., 143.

23. Ibid.

24. U.S. Department of Health and Human Services, "A Century of Women's Health," 3.

25. Ibid.

26. Boulis and Jacobs, *The Changing Face of Medicine*, 2.

27. Morgen, *Into Our Own Hands*, 129.

28. Ibid., 4–5.

29. Ibid., 122.

30. Hoffman, "Health Care Reform and Social Movements," 80.

31. Kamen, *All in My Head*, 98.

CHAPTER 5: CULTURE, CONSUMERISM, AND CHARACTER

1. "The Denver Principles," http://actupny.org/documents/Denver.html.

2. Ibid.

3. Sidell, "Adult Adjustment to Chronic Illness," 5.

4. Kerson, *Understanding Chronic Illness*, 32.

5. King, *Pink Ribbons, Inc.*, 48.

6. Elliott, *Better than Well*, xvii.

7. King, *Pink Ribbons, Inc.*, 48.

8. Elliott, *Better than Well*, 61.

9. Boehmer, *The Personal and the Political*, 12.

10. *Frontline*, "25 Years of AIDS," www.pbs.org/wgbh/pages/frontline/aids/cron/.

11. Ibid.

12. Ibid.

13. Herek, "Thinking About AIDS and Stigma," 595.

14. Ibid., 596.
15. Hoffman, "Health Care Reform," 81.
16. Boehmer, *The Personal and the Political*, 3.
17. The Body, "A History of the People With AIDS Self-Empowerment Movement," www.thebody.com/content/art31074.html?ts=pf.
18. "The Denver Principles," http://actupny.org/documents/Denver.html.
19. King, *Pink Ribbons, Inc.*, 121.
20. Ratcliff, *Women and Health*, 105.
21. Susan G. Komen for the Cure, "Breast Cancer Statistics," ww5.komen.org/Breast Cancer/Statistics.html#US.
22. Kedrowski and Sarow, *Cancer Activism: Gender, Media, and Public Policy*, 20.
23. Ibid., 21.
24. Ibid.
25. U.S. Department of Health and Human Services, "A Century of Women's Health," 31.
26. Khan, "Susan G. Komen Apologizes," http://abcnews.go.com/blogs/politics/2012/02/susan-g-komen-apologizes-for-cutting-off-planned-parenthood-funding/.
27. Kedrowski and Sarow, *Cancer Activism: Gender, Media, and Public Policy*, 24.
28. Ibid., 25.
29. Ibid.
30. Boehmer, *The Personal and the Political*, 25.
31. King, *Pink Ribbons, Inc.*, xx.
32. Ibid., 49.
33. Ibid., xxiii.
34. Susan G. Komen for the Cure, "United Against Breast Cancer," 6–9.
35. Sulik, "Enter the Komen Bandits," http://gaylesulik.com/?p=8813.
36. King, *Pink Ribbons, Inc.*, 122.
37. Rosenthal, *Everything Changes*, 7.
38. Wall, *Encounters with the Invisible*, 209.
39. Ibid., xvii.
40. Ibid.
41. Huibers and Wessely, "The Act of Diagnosis," 3.
42. Ibid.
43. Wall, *Encounters with the Invisible*, 9.
44. Strauss, "History of Chronic Fatigue Syndrome," 3.
45. Ibid., 5.
46. Klonoff, "Chronic Fatigue Syndrome," 182.
47. Centers for Disease Control and Prevention, "CFS Case Definition," www.cdc.gov/cfs/general/case_definition/index.html.
48. Wall, *Encounters with the Invisible*, 24.
49. Tuller, "Chronic Fatigue Syndrome and the CDC," www.virology.ws/2011/11/23/chronic-fatigue-syndrome-and-the-cdc-a-long-tangled-tale.

CHAPTER 6: A SLIGHT HYSTERICAL TENDENCY

1. Tuller, "Chronic Fatigue Syndrome No Longer Seen as 'Yuppie Flu,'" www
   .nytimes.com/ref/health/healthguide/esn-chronicfatigue-ess.html.
2. Morris, *The Culture of Pain*, 20.
3. American Pain Foundation, "The Problem with Pain," www.painfoundation.org
   /get-involved/problem-with-pain.html.
4. Chronic Pain Research Alliance, "Women in Pain," 3.
5. U.S. Department of Health and Human Services, "A Century of Women's
   Health," 2.
6. Society for Women's Health Research, "SWHR Timeline," www.womens
   healthresearch.org/site/PageServer?pagename=about_timeline.
7. U.S. Department of Health and Human Services, "A Century of Women's
   Health," 14.
8. Society for Women's Health Research, "SWHR Timeline."
9. Ibid.
10. U.S. Department of Health and Human Services, "A Century of Women's
    Health," 33.
11. Society for Women's Health Research, "SWHR Timeline."
12. U.S. Department of Health and Human Services, "A Century of Women's
    Health," 4.
13. Ibid., 33.
14. Ibid.
15. Hoffman and Tarzian, "The Girl Who Cried Pain," 21.
16. Ibid.
17. Chen et al., "Gender Disparity in Analgesic Treatment," 416.
18. Tuller, "Chronic Fatigue Syndrome No Longer Seen as 'Yuppie Flu.'"
19. Thernstrom, *The Pain Chronicles*, 8.
20. Medicalnewstoday.com, "More Difficult for Doctors to Diagnose Complex
    Sources of Pain," www.medicalnewstoday.com/releases/71607.php.
21. Morris, *The Culture of Pain*, 4.
22. ScienceDaily.com, "Chronic Fatigue Syndrome Not Linked to XMRV," www
    .sciencedaily.com/releases/2011/05/110504151337.htm.
23. Cohen, "Updated: In a Rare Move, *Science* without Authors' Consent Retracts
    Paper," http://news.sciencemag.org/scienceinsider/2011/12/in-a-rare-move-science
    -without-a.html#.TyM7mf8EZP4.mailto.
24. U.S. Department of Health and Human Services, "A Century of Women's
    Health," 16.
25. Marts and Resnick, Society for Women's Health Research, "Scientific Report
    Series," 1.
26. Ibid., 6.
27. Ibid.

28. Ibid.
29. Ibid., 4.
30. Fillingim et al., "Sex, Gender, and Pain," www.sciencedirect.com/science/article/pii/S1526590008009097.
31. Greenberger, "Why One Size Doesn't Fit All," www.boston.com/bostonglobe/editorial_opinion/oped/articles/2009/02/23/why_one_size_doesnt_fit_all_in_medicine/.
32. Chronic Pain Research Alliance, "Women in Pain," 9.
33. Institute of Medicine Report Brief, "Relieving Pain in America," 2–3.
34. Ibid., 3.
35. Thernstrom, *The Pain Chronicles*, 8.

CHAPTER 7: INTO THE FRAY

1. Aronowitz, "Lyme Disease," 97.
2. Ibid., 100.
3. Centers for Disease Control and Prevention, "Surveillance for Lyme Disease," www.cdc.gov/mmwr/preview/mmwrhtml/ss5710a1.htm.
4. Infectious Diseases Society of America, "Frequently Asked Questions," www.idsociety.org/lymediseasefacts.htm.
5. Fox, "The Social Life of Health Information," 5.
6. Ibid.
7. Feder et al., "A Critical Appraisal of Lyme Disease," 1428.
8. Ibid., 1422.
9. Grann, "Stalking Dr. Steere over Lyme Disease," www.nytimes.com/2001/06/17/magazine/17LYMEDISEASE.html.
10. Ibid.
11. Connecticut Attorney General's Office, "Attorney General's Investigation Reveals Flawed Lyme Disease Guidelines Process," www.ct.gov/ag/cwp/view.asp?a=2795&q=414284
12. Weintraub, *Cure Unknown*, 8.
13. Fox, "The Social Life of Health Information," 2.
14. Fox and Purcell, "Chronic Disease and the Internet 2010," 2.
15. Ibid., 3.
16. Ibid.
17. Fox, "The Social Life of Health Information," 6.
18. Ibid.
19. Ibid., 20.
20. Grann, "Stalking Dr. Steere Over Lyme Disease."
21. Ibid.
22. Tiejte, "The Worst Things People Say About Unvaccinated Kids," http://blogs.babble.com/being-pregnant/2011/07/15/the-worst-myths-about-unvaccinated-kids/.

23. *Frontline*, "Interview: Anthony S. Fauci, M.D.," www.pbs.org/wgbh/pages/front line/vaccines/interviews/fauci.html.

24. Wallace, "An Epidemic of Fear," www.wired.com/magazine/2009/10/ff_waron science/all/1.

25. *Frontline*, "Interview: Jenny McCarthy," www.pbs.org/wgbh/pages/frontline /vaccines/interviews/mccarthy.html#ixzz1UHiLAv1X.

26. Ibid.

27. Lin II, "Measles Are on the Rise," http://articles.latimes.com/2011/may/14/lo- cal/la-me-measles-20110514.

28. Offit, *Deadly Choices*, xv.

29. Ibid., 173.

30. Centers for Disease Control and Prevention, "How Many Kids Have Autism?" www.cdc.gov/ncbddd/features/counting-autism.html.

31. Wang et al., "Common Genetic Variants."

32. Parker-Pope, "Autism Risk for Siblings Higher than Expected," http://well.blogs .nytimes.com/2011/08/16/autism-risk-for-siblings-higher-than-expected/.

CHAPTER 8: PARTICIPATORY MEDICINE AND TRANSPARENCY

1. Fox, "Peer-to-Peer Healthcare," 6.

2. Ibid., 7.

3. E-Patientdave.com, "About ePatient Dave," http://epatientdave.com/about -dave.

4. KevinMD.com, "About Kevin Pho, MD," www.KevinMD.com/blog/about-kevin -md.

5. Ferguson and the e-Patient Scholars Working Group, "e-Patients," ix–x.

6. Haig, "When the Patient Is a Googler," 1, www.time.com/time/health/article /0,8599,1681838-1,00.html.

7. Trotter, "A Patient by Any Other Name," www.fredtrotter.com/2010/12/21/a -patient-by-any-other-name/.

8. Barnes et al., "Complementary and Alternative Medicine Use," 2.

9. Nakazawa, *The Autoimmune Epidemic*, 224.

10. Barnes et al., "Complementary and Alternative Medicine Use," 1.

11. Ibid., 6.

12. Ibid., 1.

13. Porter, *The Greatest Benefit to Mankind*, 689.

14. National Center for Complementary and Alternative Medicine, "About NCCAM," http://nccam.nih.gov/about/.

15. Alkon, "More Medical Schools Offer 'Alternative' Training," http://yourlife.usa today.com/health/healthyperspective/post/2011/12/More-Medical-Schools -Teaching-About-Alternative-Medicine/585142/1.

16. Novella, "The Rise of Placebo-Based Medicine," www.sciencebasedmedicine .org/index.php/the-rise-of-placebo-medicine/.

17. Nakazawa, *The Autoimmune Epidemic*, 224.

18. Barnes et al., "Complementary and Alternative Medicine Use," 6.

19. Elliott, *Better than Well*, 147.

20. Barber, "Are We Really So Miserable?" www.salon.com/life/feature/2009/08/26/barber_age_of_anxiety/index.html.

21. Ibid.

22. Angell, *The Truth About the Drug Companies*, xx.

23. Donohue, Cevasco, and Rosenthal, "A Decade of Direct-To-Consumer Advertising," 673.

24. Barber, "Are We Really So Miserable?"

25. Donohue, Cevasco, and Rosenthal, "A Decade of Direct-To-Consumer Advertising," 673.

26. News-Medical.net, "Only 15 US Pharmaceutical Ads Adhere," www.news-medical.net/news/20110819/Only-15-US-pharmaceutical-ads-adhere-to-FDA-Prescription-Drug-Advertising-Guidelines.aspx.

27. Ibid.

28. FDA.gov, "Prescription Drug Advertising: A Glossary of Terms," www.fda.gov/Drugs/ResourcesForYou/Consumers/PrescriptionDrugAdvertising/ucm072025.htm#F, "F."

29. Dreifus, "A Doctor Puts the Drug Industry Under the Microscope," 5.

30. FDAzilla.com, "About FDAzilla," http://fdazilla.com/about.aspx.

31. Gever, "Medical News: Advocacy Groups Mum on Pharma Ties," www.medpagetoday.com/PublicHealthPolicy/Ethics/24328.

CHAPTER 9: WHAT FUTURE, AT WHAT COST?

1. American Diabetes Association, "Type 1," www.diabetes.org/diabetes-basics/type1/?utm_source=WWW&utm_medium=DropDownDB&utm_content=Type1&utm_campaign=CON.

2. Roman, "Why Everyone Is So Angry," www.philly.com/philly/blogs/public_health/Why-is-everyone-so-angry-at-Paula-Deen-.html.

3. Partnership to Fight Chronic Disease, "The Growing Crisis of Chronic Disease in the United States," http://fightchronicdisease.org/resources/research.cfm.

4. Porter, *The Greatest Benefit to Mankind*, 15.

5. Ibid., 29.

6. Ibid.

7. Centers for Disease Control and Prevention, "Heart Disease Facts," www.cdc.gov/heartdisease/facts.htm.

8. American Diabetes Association, "Diabetes Statistics," www.diabetes.org/diabetes-basics/diabetes-statistics.

9. The President's Council on Fitness and Sports, "Physical Activity Facts," www.fitness.gov/resources_factsheet.htm.

10. Ibid.

11. Ibid.

12. Centers for Disease Control and Prevention, "Children and Diabetes," www.cdc .gov/diabetes/projects/cda2.htm.

13. The President's Council on Fitness and Sports, "Physical Activity Facts."

14. Centers for Disease Control and Prevention, "Childhood Obesity Facts," www .cdc.gov/healthyyouth/obesity/facts.htm.

15. Painter, "Study: US Obesity Rates Expected to Climb," http://yourlife.usatoday .com/fitness-food/diet-nutrition/story/2011-08-29/Study-Obesity-rates-pro jected-to-climb-in-US-and-UK/50180424/1?csp=ylf.

16. Pollack, "Disease of Rich Extends Its Pain," www.nytimes.com/2009/06/13/health /13gout.html?emc=eta1.

17. Ibid.

18. National Cancer Institute, "Cancer Trends Progress Report," http://progressre port.cancer.gov/doc.asp?pid=1&did=2007&mid=vcol&chid=71.

19. National Association of Chronic Disease Directors, "Health Reform, Prevention, and Chronic Disease," 2.

20. Partnership to Fight Chronic Disease, "2009 Almanac of Chronic Disease," 16.

21. Center for Science in the Public Interest, "Food Additives," http://cspinet.org /reports/chemcuisine.htm#nitrites.

22. Pollan, "Unhappy Meals," http://michaelpollan.com/articles-archive/unhappy -meals/.

23. Bittman, "Vegan Before Dinnertime," http://well.blogs.nytimes.com/2009/02/27 /vegan-before-dinnertime/.

24. Centers for Disease Control and Prevention, "Basic Statistics," www.cdc.gov/hiv /topics/surveillance/basic.htm.

25. Centers for Disease Control and Prevention, "2011 CDC Health Disparities and Inequalities Report," 3.

26. Ibid., 2.

27. Lichtenfeld, "Cancer Facts and Figures 2011," www.cancer.org/AboutUs/DrLens Blog/post/2011/06/17/Cancer-Facts-and-Figures-2011-Poverty-is-a-Carcinogen -Does-Anyone-Care.aspx.

28. American Cancer Society, "Cancer Facts and Figures 2011," 24.

29. Puhl and Heuer, "The Stigma of Obesity," 1.

30. Ibid., 4.

31. Asthma and Allergy Foundation of America, "Information About Asthma," http://www.aafa.org/display.cfm?id=9&sub=42.

32. Ibid.

33. ScienceDaily.com, "Air Pollution Alters Immune Function," www.sciencedaily .com/releases/2010/10/101005171042.htm.

34. Nakazawa, *The Autoimmune Epidemic*, 45.

35. Ibid., 51.

36. Ibid., 75.

37. Ibid., 248.

38. Harmon, "Where'd You Go with My DNA?" www.nytimes.com/2010/04/25
    /weekinreview/25harmon.html.

39. National Institutes of Health, "Stem Cell Basics," http://stemcells.nih.gov/info
    /basics/basics1.asp.

40. Jan, "Most GOP Candidates Oppose Stem Cell Funding," www.boston.com
    /news/science/articles/2011/08/07/most_gop_candidates_oppose_stem_cell
    _funding/?rss_id=Boston.com+%2F+Boston+Globe+–+National+News.

41. Henry J. Kaiser Family Foundation, "Summary of New Health Reform Law," 1.

42. Hoffman, "Health Care Reform and Social Movements," 76.

43. Ibid.

44. Ibid.

45. Ibid., 77.

46. Ibid., 78.

47. Ibid.

Bibliography

Adler, Robert E. *Medical Firsts: From Hippocrates to the Human Genome*. Hoboken, NJ: John Wiley & Sons, 2004.

Alkon, Cheryl. "More Medical Schools Offer 'Alternative' Training." http://yourlife .usatoday.com/health/healthyperspective/post/2011/12/More-Medical-Schools -Teaching-About-Alternative-Medicine/585142/1. Accessed January 29, 2012.

American Autoimmune Related Diseases Association. "Autoimmunity: A Major Women's Health Issue." www.aarda.org/women_and_autoimmunity.php. Accessed June 11, 2011.

American Cancer Society. "Cancer Facts and Figures 2011." www.cancer.org/Re search/CancerFactsFigures/CancerFactsFigures/cancer-facts-figures-2011. Accessed September 1, 2011.

American Diabetes Association. "Diabetes Statistics." www.diabetes.org/diabetes -basics/diabetes-statistics. Accessed May 19, 2010.

———. "Type 1." www.diabetes.org/diabetes-basics/type1/?utm_source=WWW& utm_medium=DropDownDB&utm_content=Type1&   utm_campaign=CON. Accessed August 31, 2011.

American Pain Foundation. "The Problem with Pain." www.painfoundation.org/get -involved/problem-with-pain.html. Accessed December 21, 2011.

Angell, Marcia, M.D. *The Truth About the Drug Companies: How They Deceive Us and What to Do About It*. New York: Random House, 2005.

Aronowitz, Robert. "Lyme Disease: The Social Construction of a New Disease and Its Social Consequences." *The Milbank Quarterly* 69, no. 1 (1991): 79–112.

Asthma and Allergy Foundation of America. "Information About Asthma, Allergies, Food Allergies, and More!" www.aafa.org/display.cfm?id=9&sub=42. Accessed September 1, 2011.

Atwood, Kimball, M.D. "Yes We Can! Abolish the NCCAM!" www.sciencebased medicine.org/index.php/yes-we-can-we-can-abolish-the-nccam/. Accessed August 19, 2011.

Barber, Charles. "Are We Really So Miserable?" www.salon.com/life/feature/2009/08
    /26/barber_age_of_anxiety/index.html. Accessed August 19, 2011.

Becker, Arielle Levin. "Blumenthal Takes Lyme Disease Fight To Senate." www.ct
    mirror.org/story/13311/blumenthal-takes-lyme-disease-fight-senate.   Accessed
    August 3, 2011.

Barnartt, Sharon, and Richard Scotch. *Disability Protests: Contentious Politics 1970–*
    1999. Washington, D.C.: Gallaudet University Press, 2001.

Barnes, Patricia M., Barbara Bloom, and Richard L. Nahin. *CDC National Health*
    Statistics Report #12. "Complementary and Alternative Medicine Use Among
    Adults and Children: United States, 2007." December 2008. http://nccam.nih
    .gov/news/camstats. Accessed August 11, 2011.

Bartholomae, David, and Anthony Pretrosky, eds. *Ways of Reading: An Anthology for*
    Writers. Boston: Bedford/St. Martin's, 2002.

Bergdolt, Klaus. *Wellbeing: A Cultural History of Healthy Living.* Malden, MA: Polity
    Press, 2008.

Bittman, Mark. "Vegan Before Dinnertime." http://well.blogs.nytimes.com/2009/02
    /27/vegan-before-dinnertime/. Accessed August 30, 2011.

Boehmer, Ulrike. *The Personal and the Political: Women's Activism in Response to*
    the Breast Cancer and AIDS Epidemics. Albany: State University of New York
    Press, 2000.

Boston Women's Health Collective and Our Bodies, Ourselves. "A Brief History and
    Reflection." www.ourbodiesourselves.org/about/jamwa4.asp. Accessed May 19,
    2011.

Boulis, Ann K., and Jerry A. Jacobs. *The Changing Face of Medicine: Women Doctors*
    and the Evolution of Health Care in America. Ithaca, NY: Cornell University
    Press, 2008.

Burton, Richard, M.D. "Big Pharma Says Your Mysterious Pain Is Real." www.salon.
    com/news/environment/mind_reader/2009/06/11/fibromyalgia/index.html.   Ac-
    cessed August 19, 2011.

Campling, Frankie, and Michael Sharpe. *Chronic Fatigue Syndrome (CFS/ME): The*
    Facts, 2nd ed. Oxford: Oxford University Press, 2008.

Center for Science in the Public Interest. "Food Additives-Food Safety." http://cspinet
    .org/reports/chemcuisine.htm#nitrites. Accessed September 1, 2011.

Centers for Disease Control and Prevention. "Basic Statistics, HIV/AIDS." www.cdc
    .gov/hiv/topics/surveillance/basic.htm. Accessed July 20, 2009.

———. "CFS Case Definition." www.cdc.gov/cfs/general/case_definition/index.html.
    Accessed March 26, 2011.

———. "Childhood Obesity Facts." www.cdc.gov/healthyyouth/obesity/facts.htm. Ac-
    cessed August 14, 2012.

———. "Children and Diabetes: More Information." www.cdc.gov/diabetes/projects
    /cda2.htm. Accessed August 30, 2011.

———. "Chronic Disease Overview." www.cdc.gov/chronicdisease/overview/index
    .htm. Accessed April 8, 2011.

———. "Heart Disease Facts." www.cdc.gov/heartdisease/facts.htm. Accessed May 19, 2010.

———. "How Many Kids Have Autism?" www.cdc.gov/ncbddd/features/counting-autism.html. Accessed August 6, 2011.

———. "Obesity and Overweight." www.cdc.gov/nchs/fastats/overwt.htm. Accessed August 30, 2011.

———. "Surveillance for Lyme Disease: 1992–2006." www.cdc.gov/mmwr/preview/mmwrhtml/ss5710a1.htm. Accessed July 27, 2011.

———. "The Tuskegee Timeline." www.cdc.gov/tuskegee/timeline.htm. Accessed May 11, 2011.

———. "2011 CDC Health Disparities and Inequalities Report." www.cdc.gov/mmwr/pdf/other/su6001.pdf. Accessed July 18, 2011.

Centers for Medicare and Medicaid Services. "Tracing the History of CMS Programs: From President Theodore Roosevelt to President Bush."

Chen, Esther H., et al.. "Gender Disparity in Analgesic Treatment of Emergency Department Patients with Acute Abdominal Pain." *Academic Emergency Medicine* (2008) 15:414–18.

"Civil Rights Chronology." Civilrights.org. The Leadership Conference on Civil and Human Rights, 2011. www.civilrights.org/resources/civilrights101/chronology.html. Accessed May 17, 2011.

Chronic Pain Research Alliance. "Women in Pain: Neglect, Dismissal and Discrimination: Analysis and Policy Recommendations." June 2011.

Cohen, Jon. "Updated: In a Rare Move, *Science* Without Authors' Consent Retracts Paper That Ties Mouse Virus to Chronic Fatigue Syndrome." http://news.sciencemag.org/scienceinsider/2011/12/in-a-rare-move-science-without-a.html#.TyM7mf8EZP4.mailto. Accessed January 27, 2012.

Conaboy, Chelsea. "Roll-back Sought on Meal Ban for Doctors." http://articles.boston.com/2011-06-16/news/29666064_1_gift-ban-meal-ban-doctors. Accessed August 20, 2011.

Connecticut Attorney General's Office. "Attorney General's Investigation Reveals Flawed Lyme Disease Guidelines Process, IDSA Agrees To Reassess Guidelines, Install Independent Arbiter." www.ct.gov/ag/cwp/view.asp?a=2795&q=414284. Accessed August 3, 2001.

Cystic Fibrosis Foundation. "About Cystic Fibrosis." www.cff.org/AboutCF. Accessed May 19, 2010.

Daaleman, Timothy, DO, MPH. "Reorganizing Medicare for Older Adults with Chronic Illness." *Journal of the American Board of Family Medicine* 19 (2006): 3. www.medscape.com/viewarticle/532512. Accessed May 12, 2011.

Deardorff, Julie. "Diabetes' Civil War." www.chicagotribune.com/health/ct-met-diabetes-rift-20101122,0,2224886,full.story. Accessed August 25, 2011.

"The Denver Principles." ACT UP/New York. http://actupny.org/documents/Denver.html. Accessed August 24, 2009.

Dolan, Amanda. "Health Communities and the Dreaded Echo Chamber." http://blog

.wegohealth.com/2011/03/21/health-communities-and-the-dreaded-echo
-chamber/. Accessed August 4, 2011.

Donohue, Julie M., Ph.D., Maria Cevasco, B.A., and Meredith B. Rosenthal, Ph.D. "A
Decade of Direct-To-Consumer Advertising of Prescription Drugs." *New England Journal of Medicine* 357, no. 7 (2007): 673–81.

Dreifus, Claudia. "A Doctor Puts the Drug Industry Under the Microscope." *New York Times,* September 14, 2004.

Edwards, Laurie. *Life Disrupted: Getting Real About Chronic Illness in Your Twenties and Thirties*. New York: Walker, 2008.

Elliott, Carl. *Better than Well: American Medicine Meets the American Dream*. New York: Norton, 2004.

E-Patientdave.com. "About ePatient Dave." http://epatientdave.com/about-dave. Accessed July 10, 2011.

Fasano et al. "Prevalence of Celiac Disease in At-Risk and Not-at-Risk Groups in the United States." *Archives of Internal Medicine* 163, no. 3 (2003): 268–92.

FDA.gov. "Prescription Drug Advertising: A Glossary of Terms." www.fda.gov/Drugs /ResourcesForYou/Consumers/PrescriptionDrugAdvertising/ucm072025.htm #F. Accessed August 21, 2011.

FDAzilla.com. "About FDAzilla." http://fdazilla.com/about.aspx. Accessed August 20, 2011.

Feder et al. "A Critical Appraisal of Lyme Disease." *New England Journal of Medicine* 357, no. 15 (2007): 1422–28.

Ferguson, Tom, M.D., and the e-Patient Scholars Working Group. "e-Patients: How They Can Help Heal Health Care." e-patients.net. 2007.

Fillingim et al. "Sex, Gender, and Pain: A Review of Recent Clinical and Experimental Findings." www.sciencedirect.com/science/article/pii/S1526590008009097. Accessed June 26, 2011.

Fowler, Wendell. "Trying to Find Common Ground." www.ss-times.com/2011/07/22 /trying-to-find-common-ground/. Accessed August 24, 2011.

Fox, Susannah. "Peer-to-Peer Healthcare." Pew Research Center's Internet & American Life Project. http://pewinternet.org/Reports/2011/P2PHealthcare.aspx. Accessed July 20, 2011.

———. "The Social Life of Health Information." Pew Research Center's Internet & American Life Project. http://pewinternet.org/Reports/2011/Social-Life-of -Health-Info.aspx. Accessed July 11, 2011.

Fox, Susannah, and Kristen Purcell. "Chronic Disease and the Internet 2010." Pew Research Center's Internet & American Life Project. http://pewinternet.org /Reports/2010/Chronic-Disease.aspx. Accessed July 12, 2011.

Frontline. "The Age of AIDS: Timeline: 25 Years of AIDS." www.pbs.org/wgbh/pages /frontline/aids/cron/. Accessed June 18, 2011.

———. "Interview: Anthony S. Fauci, M.D." www.pbs.org/wgbh/pages/frontline/vac cines/interviews/fauci.html. Accessed August 5, 2011.

———. "Interview: Jenny McCarthy." www.pbs.org/wgbh/pages/frontline/vaccines /interviews/mccarthy.html#ixzz1UHiLAv1X. Accessed August 6, 2011.

Gever, John. "Medical News: Advocacy Groups Mum on Pharma Ties." www.medpag etoday.com/PublicHealthPolicy/Ethics/24328. Accessed August 21, 2011.

Gilman, Charlotte Perkins. "The Yellow Wallpaper." www.library.csi.cuny.edu/dept /history/lavender/wallpaper.html. Accessed October 28, 2011.

Goffman, Erving. *Stigma: Notes On the Management of Spoiled Identity.* New York: Touchstone, 1986.

Grann, David. "Stalking Dr. Steere over Lyme Disease." www.nytimes.com/2001/06 /17/magazine/17LYMEDISEASE.html. Accessed August 24, 2009.

Greenberger, Phyllis. "Why One Size Doesn't Fit All." www.boston.com/bostonglobe /editorial_opinion/oped/articles/2009/02/23/why_one_size_doesnt_fit_all_in _medicine/. Accessed June 26, 2011.

Grob, Gerald. *The Deadly Truth: A History of Disease in America.* Cambridge, MA: Harvard University Press, 2002.

Habakus, Louise Kuo, and Mary Holland, eds. *Vaccine Epidemic: How Corporate Greed, Biased Science, and Coercive Government Threaten Our Human Rights, Our Health, and Our Children.* New York: Skyhorse Publishing, 2011.

Haig, Scott, M.D. "When the Patient Is a Googler." www.time.com/time/health/article /0,8599,1681838-1,00.html. Accessed July 26, 2011.

Harmon, Amy. "Where'd You Go with My DNA?" www.nytimes.com/2010/04/25 /weekinreview/25harmon.html. Accessed September 1, 2011.

Henry J. Kaiser Family Foundation. "Summary of New Health Reform Law." www.kff .org/healthreform/upload/8061.pdf. Accessed July 16, 2011.

Herek, Gregory M. "Thinking About AIDS and Stigma: A Psychologist's Perspective." *Journal of Law, Medicine & Ethics* 30 (2002): 594–607.

Hoffman, Beatrix, Ph.D. "Health Care Reform and Social Movements in the United States." Public Health Then and Now column in *American Journal of Public Health* 93, no. 1 (2003): 75–85.

Hoffman, Diane E., and Anita J. Tarzian. "The Girl Who Cried Pain: A Bias Against Women in the Treatment of Pain." *Journal of Law, Medicine and Ethics* 29 (2001): 13–27.

Huibers, Marcus, and Simon Wessely. "The Act of Diagnosis: Pros and Cons of Labeling Chronic Fatigue Syndrome" *Psychological Medicine* 36, no. 7 (2006): 1–8.

Infectious Diseases Society of America. "Frequently Asked Questions About Lyme Disease." www.idsociety.org/lymediseasefacts.htm. Accessed July 27, 2011.

Institute of Medicine Report Brief. "Relieving Pain in America: A Blueprint for Transforming Prevention, Care, Education, and Research." National Academy of Sciences, 2011.

Jan, Tracy. "Most GOP Candidates Oppose Stem Cell Funding." www.boston.com /news/science/articles/2011/08/07/most_gop_candidates_oppose_stem_cell _funding/?rss_id=Boston.com+%2F+Boston+Globe+–+National+News. Accessed September 1, 2011.

Joffe, Rosalind. "Is This Duo Doable?" http://workingwithchronicillness.com/2011/05 /is-this-duo-doable/. Accessed May 10, 2011.

Kalb, Claudia. "Stomping Through a Medical Minefield." www.thedailybeast.com

/newsweek/2008/10/24/stomping-through-a-medical-minefield.html. Accessed
   August 6, 2011.

Kamen, Paula. *All in My Head: An Epic Quest to Cure an Unrelenting, Totally Unreasonable, and Only Slightly Enlightening Headache.* Cambridge, MA: Da Capo, 2005.

Kaysen, Susanna. *The Camera My Mother Gave Me.* New York: Alfred A. Knopf,
   2001.

Kedrowski, Karen M., and Marilyn Stine Sarow. *Cancer Activism: Gender, Media,
   and Public Policy.* Urbana: University of Illinois Press, 2007.

Kelly, Kate. *Medicine Becomes a Science: 1840–1999.* New York: Infobase Publishing,
   2010.

Kennedy, Michael. *A Brief History of Disease, Science and Medicine.* Mission Viejo,
   CA: Asklepiad Press, 2004.

Kerson, Toba Schwaber, and Lawrence A. Kerson, M.D. *Understanding Chronic Illness: The Medical and Psychosocial Dimensions of Nine Diseases.* New York:
   Free Press, 1985.

KevinMD.com. "About." www.kevinmd.com/blog/about-kevin-md. Accessed January
   3, 2012.

Khan, Huma. "Susan G. Komen Apologizes for Cutting Off Planned Parenthood
   Funding."   http://abcnews.go.com/blogs/politics/2012/02/susan-g-komen-apol
   ogizes-for-cutting-off-planned-parenthood-funding/. Accessed May 16, 2012.

King, Samantha. *Pink Ribbons, Inc.: Breast Cancer and the Politics of Philanthropy.*
   Minneapolis: University of Minnesota Press, 2006.

Klonoff, David. "Chronic Fatigue Syndrome." *Clinical Infectious Diseases* 15, no. 5
   (1992): 812–23.

Kosova, Weston. "Why Health Advice on Oprah Could Make You Sick." www.thedaily
   beast.com/newsweek/2009/05/29/live-your-best-life-ever.html. Accessed August
   11, 2011.

Lepore, Jill. "The Politics of Death." *The New Yorker*, November 30, 2009, 60–69.

Lewis-Thornton, Rae. "I'm Smart, I'm Straight, and I Have AIDS." *Woman's Day*,
   May 2011, 134.

Lichtenfeld, J. Leonard, M.D. "Cancer Facts and Figures 2011: Poverty Is a Carcinogen. Does Anybody Care?" www.cancer.org/AboutUs/DrLensBlog/post/2011/06
   /17/Cancer-Facts-and-Figures-2011-Poverty-is-a-Carcinogen-Does-Anyone
   -Care.aspx. Accessed September 1, 2011.

Lin II, Rong-Gong. "Measles Are on the Rise in California." http://articles.latimes.
   com/2011/may/14/local/la-me-measles-20110514. Accessed July 25, 2011.

Long, Tony. "June 11, 1985: Karen Quinlan Dies, But the Issue Lives On." www.wired
   .com/science/discoveries/news/2008/06/dayintech_0611. Accessed May 12, 2011.

Marts, Sherry A, Ph.D., and Eileen Resnick, Ph.D. "Scientific Report Series: Understanding the Biology of Sex Differences." Society for Women's Health Research,
   May 2007.

Maugham, W. Somerset. "Sanatorium." *Sixty-Five Short Stories.* New York: Wm.
   Heineman Co., 1976.

Medicalnewstoday.com. "More Difficult for Doctors to Diagnose Complex Sources of Pain in Women Than in Men." www.medicalnewstoday.com/releases/71607.php. Accessed May 2, 2009.

Meisel, Zachary F., M.D. "Googling Symptoms: How It Can Help Patients and Doctors." www.time.com/time/health/article/0,8599,2043125,00.html. Accessed July 26, 2011.

Minnesota Statewide Independent Living Council. "A Chronology of the Disability Rights Movements." www.mnsilc.org/chronology.htm. Accessed June 22, 2010.

Morgen, Sandra. *Into Our Own Hands: The Women's Health Movement in the United States, 1969–1990*. New Brunswick, New Jersey, and London: Rutgers University Press, 2002.

Morris, David B. *The Culture of Pain*. Berkeley: University of California Press, 1991.

———. "How To Speak Postmodern: Medicine, Illness, and Cultural Change," *The Hastings Center Report*, November–December 2000, 7–16.

Nakazawa, Donna Jackson. *The Autoimmune Epidemic: Bodies Gone Haywire in a World out of Balance—and the Cutting-Edge Science that Promises Hope*. New York: Touchstone, 2008.

National Association of Chronic Disease Directors. "Health Reform, Prevention, and Chronic Disease: The Next Steps," April 2010. www.diseasechronic.org/files /public/PatientProtectionandAffordableCareAct.pdf. Accessed July 16, 2011.

National Cancer Institute. "Cancer Trends Progress Report: Prevention." http:// progressreport.cancer.gov/doc.asp?pid=1&did=2007&mid=vcol&chid=71. Accessed September 1, 2011.

National Capital Poison Center. "Vaccines Do Not Cause Autism." www.poison.org /current/autism%20and%20vaccines.htm. Accessed December 28, 2011.

National Center for Complementary and Alternative Medicine. "About NCCAM." http://nccam.nih.gov/about/. Accessed August 12, 2011.

National Hospice and Palliative Care Organization. "NHPCO Facts and Figures: Hospice Care in America." 2011.

National Institutes of Health. "The 1971 National Cancer Act: Investment in the Future." www.nih.gov/news/pr/mar97/nci-26c.htm. Accessed May 10, 2011.

———. "Stem Cell Basics: Introduction." http://stemcells.nih.gov/info/basics/basics1 .asp. Accessed September 1, 2011.

National Institutes of Health, Office of History. "Timeline of Laws Related to the Protection of Human Subjects." http://history.nih.gov/about/timelines_laws _human.html#1949. Accessed June 21, 2010.

National Organization for Women. "NOW FAQs." www.now.org/organization/faq .html#found. Accessed June 13, 2011.

News-Medical.net. "Only 15 US Pharmaceutical Ads Adhere to FDA Prescription Drug Advertising Guidelines." www.news-medical.net/news/20110819/Only-15 -US-pharmaceutical-ads-adhere-to-FDA-Prescription-Drug-Advertising -Guidelines.aspx. Accessed August 20, 2011.

Novella, Steven, M.D. "The Rise of Placebo-Based Medicine." www.sciencebased medicine.org/index.php/the-rise-of-placebo-medicine/. Accessed August 13, 2011.

NPR.org. "A Look Back at 'Section 504,'" www.npr.org/programs/wesun/features /2002/504/. Accessed June 8, 2011.

———. "Remembering the Tuskegee Experiment." www.npr.org/programs/morning/ features/2002/jul/tuskegee/. Accessed May 11, 2011.

Offit, Paul A., M.D. *Deadly Choices: How the Anti-Vaccine Movement Threatens Us All*. New York: Basic Books, 2011.

Painter, Kim. "Gluten-free Diets Gaining in Popularity." www.usatoday.com/news /health/painter/2008-08-17-gluten_N.htm. Accessed August 30, 2011.

———. "Study: US Obesity Rates Expected to Climb." http://yourlife.usatoday.com /fitness-food/diet-nutrition/story/2011-08-29/Study-Obesity-rates-projected-to -climb-in-US-and-UK/50180424/1?csp=ylf. Accessed September 1, 2011.

Parker-Pope, Tara. "Autism Risk for Siblings Higher than Expected." http://well.blogs .nytimes.com/2011/08/16/autism-risk-for-siblings-higher-than-expected/. Accessed August 21, 2011.

Partnership to Fight Chronic Disease. "Facing the Issues: About the Crisis." http:// fightchronicdisease.org/issues/about.cfm. Accessed May 17, 2010.

———. "The Growing Crisis of Chronic Disease in the United States." http:// fightchronicdisease.org/resources/research.cfm. Accessed November 13, 2009.

———. "2009 Almanac of Chronic Disease: The Impact of Chronic Disease on U.S. Health and Prosperity." www.fightchronicdisease.org/resources/almanac -chronic-disease-0. Accessed September 1, 2011.

Pollack, Andrew. "Disease of Rich Extends its Pain to the Middle Class." www.ny times.com/2009/06/13/health/13gout.html?emc=eta1. Accessed August 29, 2011.

Pollan, Michael. "Unhappy Meals." http://michaelpollan.com/articles-archive/unhappy -meals/. Accessed August 30, 2011.

Porter, Roy. *Blood and Guts: A Short History of Medicine*. New York: W.W. Norton & Company, 2004.

———. *The Greatest Benefit to Mankind: A Medical History of Humanity*. New York: W.W. Norton & Company, 1999.

President's Council on Fitness and Sports. "Physical Activity Facts." www.fitness.gov /resources_factsheet.htm. Accessed August 30, 2011.

Price, Bill. "Johnson & Johnson: A View on the Facebook Policy Change." http://jnjbtw .com/2011/08/johnson-johnson-%E2%80%93-a-view-on-the-facebook-policy -change/. Accessed August 21, 2011.

Puhl, Rebecca M., and Chelsea A. Heuer. "The Stigma of Obesity: A Review and Update." Yale Rudd Center for Food Policy and Obesity, 2009. www.yaleruddcenter .org/resources/upload/docs/ ... /WeightBiasStudy.pdf. Accessed September 1, 2011.

Quigley, James. "Hospitals and the Civil Rights Act of 1964." *Journal of the National Medical Association* 57, no. 6 (1965): 455–59.

Rao, Jaya K., MD, MHS. "Looking Back and Looking Forward." *Preventing Chronic Disease* 5, no. 1 (2008). www.cdc.gov/pcd/issues/2008/jan/07_0179.htm. Accessed January 19, 2010.

Ratcliff, Kathryn Stother. *Women and Health: Power, Technology, Inequality and Conflict in a Gendered World.* Boston: Allyn and Bacon, 2002.

Raymond, Joan. "The Stigma of Illness: Getting Sick Is Bad Enough, but Being Judged for It May Be Even Worse." *Woman's Day*, May 2011, 133–38.

Roberts, Dean W., M.D., M.P.H. "The Commission on Chronic Illness." *Public Health Reports (1896–1970)* 69, no. 3 (1954): 295–99.

Roman, Leah. "Why Everyone Is So Angry at Paula Deen." www.philly.com/philly /blogs/public_health/Why-is-everyone-so-angry-at-Paula-Deen-.html. Accessed May 30, 2012.

Rosenbloom, Stephanie. "Calorie Data To Be Posted at Most Chains." www.nytimes .com/2010/03/24/business/24menu.html. Accessed September 1, 2011.

Rosenthal, Kairol. "Happy Birthday to You." http://everythingchangesbook.com/kairol /affordable-care-act-on-year-anniversary. Accessed September 1, 2011.

———. "Using Sex To Sell Breast Cancer?" http://everythingchangesbook.com/kairol /rethink-breast-cancer. Accessed November 15, 2009.

Rothman, David J. *Strangers at the Bedside: A History of How Law and Bioethics Transformed Medical Decision Making.* New York: Walter de Gruyter, 2003.

Ruzek, Sheryl. "Transforming Doctor-Patient Relationships." *Journal of Health Services Research and Policy* 12, no. 3 (2007): 181–82.

Sampson, Wallace, M.D. "Why the National Center for Complementary and Alternative Medicine (NCCAM) Should Be Defunded." www.quackwatch.org/01Quack eryRelatedTopics/nccam.html. Accessed August 13, 2011.

ScienceDaily.com. "Air Pollution Alters Immune Function, Worsens Asthma Symptoms, Study Finds." www.sciencedaily.com/releases/2010/10/101005171042.htm. Accessed September 1, 2011.

———. "Chronic Fatigue Syndrome Not Linked to XMRV, Comprehensive Study Finds." www.sciencedaily.com/releases/2011/05/110504151337.htm. Accessed June 26, 2011.

Sidell, Nancy L. "Adult Adjustment to Chronic Illness: A Review of the Literature." *Health & Social Work* 22, no. 1 (1997): 5–11.

Skambis, Kathleen. "I Had Lung Cancer and Never Smoked a Day in My Life." *Woman's Day*, May 2011, 136–37.

Skloot, Rebecca. *The Immortal Life of Henrietta Lacks.* New York: Crown, 2010.

Society for Women's Health Research. "SWHR Timeline." www.womenshealthresearch .org/site/PageServer?pagename=about_timeline. Accessed February 12, 2011.

Sontag, Susan. *Illness as Metaphor and AIDS and Its Metaphors.* New York: Picador, 2001.

Strauss, Stephen. "History of Chronic Fatigue Syndrome." *Reviews of Infectious Diseases: Considerations in the Design of Studies of Chronic Fatigue Syndrome* 13, no. 1 (1991): S2–S7.

Sulik, Gayle. "Enter the Komen Bandits: Racing with a Message for BC METS." http://gaylesulik.com/?p=8813. Accessed June 23, 2011.

Susan G. Komen for the Cure. "Breast Cancer Statistics." ww5.komen.org/Breast Cancer/Statistics.html#US. Accessed August 11, 2012.

Susan G. Komen for the Cure. "United Against Breast Cancer: 2009–2010 Annual Report." 2010.

The Body. "A History of the People With AIDS Self-Empowerment Movement." www.thebody.com/content/art31074.html?ts=pf. Accessed August 24, 2009.

Thernstrom, Melanie. *The Pain Chronicles*. New York: Farrar, Straus and Giroux, 2010.

Tiejte, Kate. "The Worst Things People Say About Unvaccinated Kids." http://blogs.babble.com/being-pregnant/2011/07/15/the-worst-myths-about-unvaccinated-kids/. Accessed August 6, 2011.

Torres, Christian. "Drug Companies Lose Protection on Facebook, Some Decide to Close Pages." www.washingtonpost.com/national/health-science/pharmaceutical-companies-lose-protections-on-facebook-decide-to-close-pages/2011/07/22/gIQATQGFBJ_story.html. Accessed August 21, 2011.

Trotter, Fred. "A Patient by Any Other Name." www.fredtrotter.com/2010/12/21/a-patient-by-any-other-name/. Accessed August 11, 2011.

Tuller, David. "Chronic Fatigue Syndrome and the CDC: A Long, Tangled Tale." www.virology.ws/2011/11/23/chronic-fatigue-syndrome-and-the-cdc-a-long-tangled-tale. Accessed August 11, 2012.

———. "Chronic Fatigue Syndrome No Longer Seen as 'Yuppie Flu.'" *New York Times*. www.nytimes.com/ref/health/healthguide/esn-chronicfatigue-ess.html. Accessed May 2, 2009.

United States Department of Health and Human Services. "The Great Pandemic: The United States in 1918–1919." http://1918.pandemicflu.gov/the_pandemic/04.htm. Accessed June 25, 2011.

United States Department of Health and Human Services, Office on Women's Health. "A Century of Women's Health." 2002.

University of California Berkeley, The Disability Rights and Independent Living Movement. "Introduction." http://bancroft.berkeley.edu/collections/drilm/introduction.html. Accessed June 22, 2010.

———. "Timeline." http://bancroft.berkeley.edu/collections/drilm/resources/timeline.html. Accessed June 2, 2011.

Wall, Dorothy. *Encounters with the Invisible: Unseen Illness, Controversy, and Chronic Fatigue Syndrome*. Dallas: Southern Methodist University Press, 2005.

Wallace, Amy. "An Epidemic of Fear: How Panicked Parents Skipping Shots Endangers Us All." www.wired.com/magazine/2009/10/ff_waronscience/all/1. Accessed July 24, 2011.

Wang, Kai, et al. "Common Genetic Variants on 5p14.1 Associate with Autism Spectrum." *Nature* 459 (2009): 528–33.

Weintraub, Pamela. *Cure Unknown: Inside the Lyme Epidemic.* New York: St. Martin's Press, 2008.

Wendell, Susan. "Unhealthy Disabled: Treating Chronic Illness as Disabilities." *Hypatia* 16, no. 4 (2001): 17–33.

Womenshealth.gov. "Infertility: Frequently Asked Questions." www.womenshealth.gov/faq/infertility.cfm#b. Accessed June 11, 2011.

Woodward, Roslyn, and Dorothy Broom. "Diagnosis in Chronic Illness: Disabling or Enabling—the Case of Chronic Fatigue Syndrome." *Journal of the Royal Society of Medicine* 89 (1995): 325–29.

Index

Understanding Chronic Illness
(Toba Schwaber), 88
Unger, Elizabeth, 107
unhealthy disabled, 52
universal health care, 60
urbanization, 18–19
U.S. Department of Health, Education,
and Welfare, 59, 63
U.S. Department of Health and Human
Services, 82
U.S. Public Health Service, 40
USA Today, 160

vaccination, 22
vaccines
controversy surrounding, 147–157
National Vaccine Injury Compensation
Program, 151
polio, 26
validity (of information), 166
viral petitions, 155
virtual advocacy, 143–157

Wall, Dorothy, 10, 105
Wallace, Amy, 149
Weintraub, Karen, 150
Weintraub, Pamela, 135
Wendell, Susan, 52, 65

White, Ryan, 87, 92
Whitman, Sarah, 74, 114
WHO (World Health Organization), 26, 91
Winfrey, Oprah, 149
Wired, 149
women
and "emotional" vs. "real" pain, 115
in Middle Ages, 19–20
pain in men vs., 110
and plight of the female patient, 76–84
stereotyping of, 84
Women's Equity Action League, 82
women's health advocacy, 84–86
women's health movement, 69–86
World AIDS Day, 87
World Health Organization (WHO),
26, 91
World Medical Association, 40
Wright, Joe, 54, 64–65, 76, 92, 94–96,
204–205

XMRV retrovirus, 124

The Yellow Wallpaper (Charlotte Perkins
Gillman), 70–71
Y-ME, 97
YouTube, 178
yuppie flu, 87

A Note on the Author

Laurie Edwards is a graduate of Georgetown University and received her M.F.A. in nonfiction writing from Emerson College. She is a patient advocate and lifelong patient with multiple chronic illnesses, including primary ciliary dyskinesia (PCD), a rare genetic lung disease, and autoimmune diseases. Her first book, *Life Disrupted: Getting Real About Chronic Illness in Your Twenties and Thirties*, was named one of 2008's Best Consumer Health books by *Library Journal*. She has written for the *Boston Globe*, *Boston Globe Magazine*, *Glamour*, and many other outlets, and her health blog, www.achronicdose.com, has been featured in *Wired* and on numerous other blogs and websites. Edwards teaches health science writing at Northeastern University and lives outside Boston, Massachusetts, with her husband, daughter, and rescue dog.